Current Challenges and Advances in Cataract Surgery

Current Challenges and Advances in Cataract Surgery

Editor

Nobuyuki Shoji

MDPI • Basel • Beijing • Wuhan • Barcelona • Belgrade • Manchester • Tokyo • Cluj • Tianjin

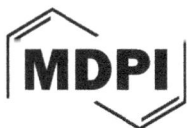

Editor
Nobuyuki Shoji
Kitasato University School of Medicine
Japan

Editorial Office
MDPI
St. Alban-Anlage 66
4052 Basel, Switzerland

This is a reprint of articles from the Special Issue published online in the open access journal *Journal of Clinical Medicine* (ISSN 2077-0383) (available at: https://www.mdpi.com/journal/jcm/special_issues/cataract_surgery_research).

For citation purposes, cite each article independently as indicated on the article page online and as indicated below:

LastName, A.A.; LastName, B.B.; LastName, C.C. Article Title. *Journal Name* **Year**, *Volume Number*, Page Range.

ISBN 978-3-0365-6277-3 (Hbk)
ISBN 978-3-0365-6278-0 (PDF)

© 2023 by the authors. Articles in this book are Open Access and distributed under the Creative Commons Attribution (CC BY) license, which allows users to download, copy and build upon published articles, as long as the author and publisher are properly credited, which ensures maximum dissemination and a wider impact of our publications.
The book as a whole is distributed by MDPI under the terms and conditions of the Creative Commons license CC BY-NC-ND.

Contents

Preface to "Current Challenges and Advances in Cataract Surgery" vii

Wei-Cheng Chang, Cho-Hao Lee, Shih-Hwa Chiou, Chen-Chung Liao and Chao-Wen Cheng
Proteomic Analysis of Aqueous Humor Proteins in Association with Cataract Risks: Diabetes and Smoking
Reprinted from: *J. Clin. Med.* **2021**, *10*, 5731, doi:10.3390/jcm10245731 1

Yoshihiko Iida, Kimiya Shimizu and Nobuyuki Shoji
Development of a New Method for Calculating Intraocular Lens Power after Myopic Laser In Situ Keratomileusis by Combining the Anterior–Posterior Ratio of the Corneal Radius of the Curvature with the Double-K Method
Reprinted from: *J. Clin. Med.* **2022**, *11*, 522, doi:10.3390/jcm11030522 17

Young-Sik Yoo and Woong-Joo Whang
Conditional Process Analysis for Effective Lens Position According to Preoperative Axial Length
Reprinted from: *J. Clin. Med.* **2022**, *11*, 1469, doi:10.3390/jcm11061469 27

Otman Sandali, Rachid Tahiri Joutei Hassani, Ashraf Armia Balamoun, Mohamed El Sanharawi and Vincent Borderie
Facilitating Role of the 3D Viewing System in Tilted Microscope Positions for Cataract Surgery in Patients Unable to Lie Flat
Reprinted from: *J. Clin. Med.* **2022**, *11*, 1865, doi:10.3390/jcm11071865 39

Barbara S. Brunner, Nikolaus Luft, Siegfried G. Priglinger, Mehdi Shajari, Wolfgang J. Mayer and Stefan Kassumeh
Saving of Time Using a Software-Based versus a Manual Workflow for Toric Intraocular Lens Calculation and Implantation
Reprinted from: *J. Clin. Med.* **2022**, *11*, 2907, doi:10.3390/jcm11102907 45

Yueh-Ling Chen, Christy Pu, Ken-Kuo Lin, Jiahn-Shing Lee, Laura Liu and Chiun-Ho Hou
A Comparison of Visual Quality and Contrast Sensitivity between Patients with Scleral-Fixated and In-Bag Intraocular Lenses
Reprinted from: *J. Clin. Med.* **2022**, *11*, 2917, doi:10.3390/jcm11102917 53

Yoshihiko Iida, Kimiya Shimizu and Nobuyuki Shoji
Reply to Cione et al. Comment on "Iida et al. Development of a New Method for Calculating Intraocular Lens Power after Myopic Laser In Situ Keratomileusis by Combining the Anterior–Posterior Ratio of the Corneal Radius of the Curvature with the Double-K Method. *J. Clin. Med.* 2022, *11*, 522"
Reprinted from: *J. Clin. Med.* **2022**, *11*, 2708, doi:10.3390/jcm11102708 63

Mario Damiano Toro, Serena Milan, Daniele Tognetto, Robert Rejdak, Ciro Costagliola, Sandrine Anne Zweifel, Chiara Posarelli, Michele Figus, Magdalena Rejdak, Teresio Avitabile, Adriano Carnevali and Rosa Giglio
Intraoperative Anterior Segment Optical Coherence Tomography in the Management of Cataract Surgery: State of the Art
Reprinted from: *J. Clin. Med.* **2022**, *11*, 3867, doi:10.3390/jcm11133867 67

Roman Lischke, Walter Sekundo, Rainer Wiltfang, Martin Bechmann, Thomas C. Kreutzer, Siegfried G. Priglinger, Martin Dirisamer and Nikolaus Luft
IOL Power Calculations and Cataract Surgery in Eyes with Previous Small Incision Lenticule Extraction
Reprinted from: *J. Clin. Med.* **2022**, *11*, 4418, doi:10.3390/jcm11154418 81

Miki Omoto, Kaoruko Sugawara, Hidemasa Torii, Erisa Yotsukura, Sachiko Masui, Yuta Shigeno, Yasuyo Nishi and Kazuno Negishi
Investigating the Prediction Accuracy of Recently Updated Intraocular Lens Power Formulas with Artificial Intelligence for High Myopia
Reprinted from: *J. Clin. Med.* **2022**, *11*, 4848, doi:10.3390/jcm11164848 91

Anna Dołowiec-Kwapisz, Halina Piotrowska and Marta Misiuk-Hojło
Evaluation of Visual and Patient—Reported Outcomes, Spectacle Dependence after Bilateral Implantation with a Non-Diffractive Extended Depth of Focus Intraocular Lens Compared to Other Intraocular Lenses
Reprinted from: *J. Clin. Med.* **2022**, *11*, 5246, doi:10.3390/jcm11175246 99

Majid Moshirfar, Kathryn M. Durnford, Jenna L. Jensen, Daniel P. Beesley, Telyn S. Peterson, Ines M. Darquea, Yasmyne C. Ronquillo and Phillip C. Hoopes
Accuracy of Six Intraocular Lens Power Calculations in Eyes with Axial Lengths Greater than 28.0 mm
Reprinted from: *J. Clin. Med.* **2022**, *11*, 5947, doi:10.3390/jcm11195947 113

Wei-Tsun Chen, Yu-Yen Chen and Man-Chen Hung
Dry Eye Following Femtosecond Laser-Assisted Cataract Surgery: A Meta-Analysis
Reprinted from: *J. Clin. Med.* **2022**, *11*, 6228, doi:10.3390/jcm11216228 123

Preface to "Current Challenges and Advances in Cataract Surgery"

I have organized this Special Issue to discuss appropriate IOL formulas, the proper use of special intraocular lenses, and the current status of cataract surgery for special ocular situations, and invited research papers. We received a number of submissions and, through detailed peer review, we were able to carefully select excellent research papers for publication.

Chang et al. collected aqueous humor during cataract surgery and, by examining this, showed that the alpha-2-HS-glycoprotein, called fetuin-a, could be a potential aqueous 35 biomarker associated with DM and smoking, which are cataract risk factors.

The new IOL power calculation formula for post-LASIK eyes by Iida et al. is considered a very useful study in the context of the increasing number of post-refractive cataract surgery patients. The comments of Cione et al. on this paper and the response of Iida et al. must also be of interest to the reader. Similarly, we believe that the IOL power calculation after SMILE is also information that will be needed in the future. Lischke et al. reported that the ray-tracking method showed superior predictability in IOL power calculation over empirically optimized IOL power calculation formulae that were originally intended for use after Excimer-based keratorefractive procedures. The improvement in postoperative visual quality is an important and unavoidable issue in current cataract surgery, and the report by Brunner et al. on the more accurate calculation and insertion of toric IOLs is very informative. A problem that has been vexing many surgeons is IOL calculation in highly myopic or long-axis eyes. The reports of Moshirfar et al. and Omoto et al. must be of great help to surgeons. The study by Yoo et al. on the most effective lens position according to preoperative axis length is also very interesting.

The surgical method demonstrated by Sandali et al., which applies the 3D system to patients who have difficulty lying supine during surgery, should be a bright light for patients and their families who have given up on surgery. The review by Toro et al. shows that intraoperative anterior segment, OCT, is not only useful for novel surgeons, but is also a useful tool for education on and management of the complicated cases of cataract surgery for expert surgeons. Scleral-fixated occurs when in-the-bag IOL fixation fails for some reason, but it is also possible that the IOL fixation is unstable, resulting in reduced visual function. Chen YL et al. provide an in-depth discussion of this. The study by Dołowiec-Kwapisz et al. of the spectacle dependence of EDOF and the photic phenomenon provides important information when recommending this type of IOL to patients. A thorough preoperative explanation of the degree of dependence on spectacle would avoid unnecessary problems due to decreased postoperative satisfaction. FLAC is attracting attention as the next generation of cataract surgery, but various problems have been pointed out. Dry eyes are one of them. Chen WT et al. point out this problem by conducting a meta-analysis. As mentioned above, the papers discuss a variety of topics, from preoperative to intraoperative and postoperative, and I believe that this is a very interesting Special Issue.

Finally, I would like to express my sincere respect to all the authors, who submitted excellent papers, and to the reviewers who took the trouble to review them.

Nobuyuki Shoji
Editor

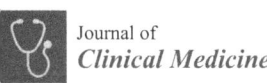

Article

Proteomic Analysis of Aqueous Humor Proteins in Association with Cataract Risks: Diabetes and Smoking

Wei-Cheng Chang [1,2], Cho-Hao Lee [3], Shih-Hwa Chiou [4,5,6,7], Chen-Chung Liao [8] and Chao-Wen Cheng [1,9,10,*]

1. Graduate Institute of Clinical Medicine, College of Medicine, Taipei Medical University, Taipei 11031, Taiwan; cwc761229@gmail.com
2. Department of Ophthalmology, Taoyuan General Hospital, Ministry of Health and Welfare, Taoyuan 33004, Taiwan
3. Division of Hematology and Oncology, Department of Internal Medicine, Tri-Service General Hospital, National Defense Medical Center, Taipei 114202, Taiwan; drleechohao@gmail.com
4. Department of Medical Research, Taipei Veterans General Hospital, Taipei 11217, Taiwan; shchiou@vghtpe.gov.tw
5. School of Medicine, National Yang-Ming University, Taipei 11221, Taiwan
6. Institute of Pharmacology, National Yang-Ming University, Taipei 11221, Taiwan
7. Genomic Research Center, Academia Sinica, Taipei 11529, Taiwan
8. Metabolomics-Proteomics Research Center, National Yang Ming Chiao Tung University, Taipei 11221, Taiwan; ccliao@ym.edu.tw
9. Traditional Herbal Medicine Research Center, Taipei Medical University Hospital, Taipei Medical University, Taipei 11031, Taiwan
10. Cell Physiology and Molecular Image Research Center, Wan Fang Hospital, Taipei Medical University, Taipei 11031, Taiwan
* Correspondence: ccheng@tmu.edu.tw

Abstract: Cataracts are one of the most common eye diseases that can cause blindness. Discovering susceptibility factors in the proteome that contribute to cataract development would be helpful in gaining new insights in the molecular mechanisms of the cataract process. We used label-free nanoflow ultra-high-performance liquid chromatography–tandem mass spectrometry to compare aqueous humor protein expressions in cataract patients with different cataract risk factors such as diabetes mellitus (DM) and smoking and in controls (with cataract) without risk exposure. Eight patients with diabetes and who smoked (with double risk factors), five patients with diabetes and five patients who smoked (both with a single risk factor), and nine aged-matched cataract controls patients (non-risk exposure) were enrolled. In total, 136 aqueous humor proteins were identified, of which only alpha-2-Heremans–Schmid (HS)-glycoprotein was considered to be significantly risk-associated because it was differentially expressed in these three groups and exhibited increased expression with increasing risk factors. Significant changes in the aqueous humor level of alpha-2-HS-glycoprotein between DM and control samples and between smoking and control samples were confirmed using ELISA. The alpha-2-HS-glycoprotein, called fetuin-a, could be a potential aqueous biomarker associated with DM and smoking, which were cataract risk factors.

Keywords: aqueous humor; label free; cataract; risk factor; proteomics; alpha-2-HS-glycoprotein; fetuin-A

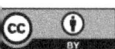

1. Introduction

In developed countries, cataracts are one of the most common causes of blindness [1]. They are classified by cause as age-related cataracts, pediatric cataracts, and cataracts secondary to other causes. As shown by many studies, age is the biggest risk factor [2,3]. Considering the location of opacification within the lens, cataracts are divided into three major types: nuclear, cortical, and posterior subcapsular cataracts. Cataract development can be caused by many other risk factors, including environmental factors and genetic changes [4]. Diabetes mellitus (DM), long-term use of corticosteroids, cigarette smoking, prolonged exposure to ultraviolet light, and alcohol abuse are well-known risk factors [2]. Cigarette smoking is a risk factor for nuclear and posterior subcapsular cataracts [4]. DM was identified as a common cause of posterior subcapsular and cortical cataracts [5,6]. Increased age is a risk factor for the development of all types of cataracts. Throughout life, a high myopia of over −6.0 D is associated with nuclear cataracts and posterior subcapsular cataracts [7]. Other causes of cataracts include mechanical trauma, chemical injury, electrical injury, radiation, and certain medications. However, the underlying cataractogenic mechanisms of cataract development are still not well documented, with many still being investigated. Proteomics analysis is an extensively used technique to discover changes in protein levels in tissues and cells. Recent proteomic studies in cataract disease of the human aqueous humor (AH) revealed multiple proteins of interest in patients [8–12]. Ji et al. [13] used isobaric tags for the relative and absolute quantitation (iTRAQ) methodology to compare AH protein profiles among high myopia, glaucoma, and vitrectomy surgery patients, and controls. They identified multiple candidate protein biomarkers associated with cataract development in each group. Furthermore, Kim et al. [14] analyzed the aqueous proteome from age-related macular degeneration (AMD) patients and non-AMD cataract controls to identify novel pathogenic proteins that are useful as potential clinical biomarkers. The differential expressions of three proteins were reported in the AH of AMD patients compared with those of cataract controls. Those studies used a good model that inspired a new idea for us of using proteomics to discuss different risk factors of cataract formation. To our knowledge, there has been no previous investigation of different cataract risk factors by comparing proteomic evidence. We used proteomics to discover the pathogenesis of different cataract risks and to possibly identify candidate biomarker proteins identified in patients predisposed to this condition. In this study, we employed Nanoflow ultra-high-performance liquid chromatography–tandem mass spectrometry (n-UPLC-MS/MS) to examine the protein compositions of aqueous solutions obtained from human cataract eyes of patients who had a single risk factor of either DM or cigarette smoking, those who had double risk factors of DM and cigarette smoking, and aged-matched cataract controls (with neither risk factor). This sensitive proteomics approach could help examine the underlying pathophysiology of cataract formation using relatively scarce amounts of aqueous samples, thereby favoring the methodological approach for this investigation. This study may reveal valuable insights into the molecular changes in the AH in the course of cataract pathogenesis.

2. Materials and Methods

2.1. Subjects

The study protocol was approved by the Medical Ethics and Institutional Review Board of Taoyuan General Hospital, Ministry of Health and Welfare (TYGH109009) (Taoyuan, Taiwan), and conducted as per the tenets of the Declaration of Helsinki. All study participants provided written informed consent before their enrollment, and the nature and possible consequences of the study were explained to them. Human AH samples from treatment-naive patients with a single risk factor ($n = 10$) of DM ($n = 5$) or cigarette smoking ($n = 5$), double risk factors ($n = 8$) of DM combined with cigarette smoking, and aged-matched cataract controls with neither risk factor ($n = 9$) were collected while patients were undergoing cataract surgery at Taoyuan General Hospital. The diagnostic criterion for cataracts was defined with a slit lamp with no other ocular diseases, trauma, or previous intraocular operation history. The presence of type 2 diabetes was defined as any one or more of the following: (1) having had a diagnosis of type 2 diabetes that was confirmed by a physician (ICD10: E11); (2) self-report of a diabetes diagnosis and use of hypoglycemic medications; (3) a fasting glucose level of ≥ 126 mg/dL; (4) a 2 h post-challenge plasma glucose level of ≥ 200 mg/dL. All subjects were included as cases of type 2 diabetes within a follow-up time of five years. A cigarette smoking history was obtained from all patients. Their cigarette consumption varied with a mean duration of more than 20 years. Data on control eyes were collected from senior cataract patients who were free from other ocular or systemic diseases. In these three groups, inclusion criteria were cataract patients aged older than 55 years. Exclusion criteria were a history of any systemic or ocular disorder or condition including ocular surgery, trauma, or disease. Best corrected visual acuity (BCVA) was measured as the logarithm of the minimum angle of resolution (logMAR).

2.2. AH Sample Collection

AH samples were obtained from patients during the implantation of phakic intraocular lenses. To avoid hemorrhaging and ocular surface contamination, a sample was collected using a 1 mL tuberculin syringe with a 30 gauge needle at the limbus before any other entry into the eye under a surgical microscope. Note that 50–100 µL of AH was collected from each patient by anterior chamber paracentesis. Undiluted AH samples were collected and stored at $-80\ ^\circ C$ within 24 h until preparation was initiated.

2.3. n-UPLC-MS/MS

Protein concentrations of AH samples were determined by a dye-binding method based on the Bradford assay (Bio-Rad Laboratories, Richmond, CA, USA) (Table 1), and samples were further diluted in 1× phosphate-buffered saline (PBS) to a final concentration of 0.1 µg/µL. Samples were prepared as per the SMART digestion kit protocol from ThermoFisher Scientific (Waltham, MA, USA) and cleaned up using solid-phase extraction (SPE) plates from ThermoFisher. The resulting peptides collected from the filters were dried in a vacuum centrifuge and stored at $-80\ ^\circ C$. Then, 50 µL of diluted AH samples was resuspended in 0.1% formic acid and analyzed by n-UPLC-MS/MS. Tryptic peptides were loaded into an LTQ-Orbitrap mass spectrometer with a nanoelectrospray ionization source (Thermo Electron, MA, USA) connected to a nanoACQUITY UPLC system (Waters, MA, USA). Peptide samples were separated on a 25 cm × 75 µm BEH130 C18 column (Waters) with a 0–95% segmented gradient of 3–40% B for 168 min, 40–95% B for 2 min, and 95% B for 10 min at a flow rate of 0.5 µL/min. Mobile phase A was 0.1% formic acid in water, while mobile phase B was 0.1% formic acid in acetonitrile. The mass spectrometer was set to the data-dependent acquisition method (isolation width: 1.5 Da). As per the data-dependent acquisition method, the first ten most intensively charged peptide ions were selected and fragmented using a collision-induced dissociation (CID) method (Figure 1).

Table 1. Demographic characteristics of enrolled patients with a single risk factor, those with Double risk factors, and cataract controls.

	Cataract Control	Single Risk	Double Risks	p Value [#]
Gender				0.003
Female	7 (77.8%)	3 (30.0%)	0 (0.0%)	
Male	2 (22.2%)	7 (70.0%)	8 (100.0%)	
Protein (µg/µL)	0.22 ± 0.06	0.36 ± 0.21	0.34 ± 0.11	0.049
Age (years)	74.00 ± 5.72	72.30 ± 10.14	69.38 ± 9.87	0.390
VA (logMAR)	0.41 ± 0.12	0.38 ± 0.14	0.27 ± 0.20	0.360
AXL (mm)	23.48 ± 0.59	24.02 ± 1.24	23.69 ± 0.95	0.552
Smoking		5		
Diabetes mellitus (DM)		5		
Smoking + DM			8	

[#] By Fisher's exact test, Wilcoxon test, or Kruskal–Wallis test.

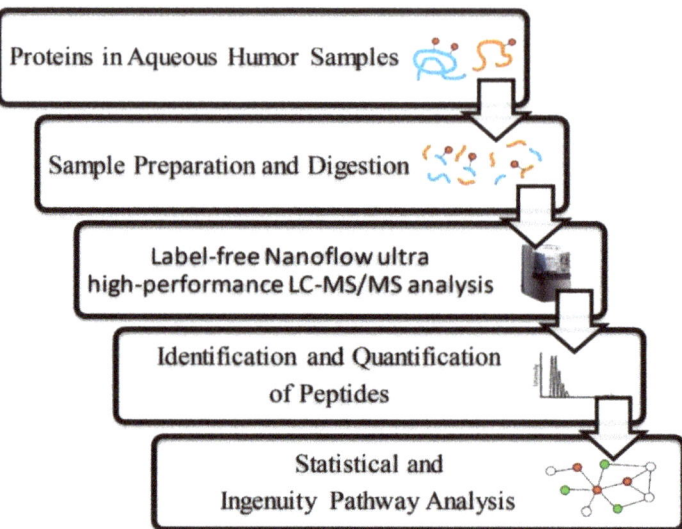

Figure 1. Label-free Nanoflow UHPLC-MS/MS analytical workflow for the proteomic analysis of human aqueous humor. Samples were digested using trypsin and were analyzed using an LTQ-Orbitrap DiscoveryTM hybrid mass spectrometer (Thermo Electron). Proteins were identified and quantified using the SEQUEST algorithm followed by analysis using Xcalibur 2.0 SR1 (Thermo Electron).

2.4. Protein Identification

Then, the acquired MS/MS raw data files were applied to search against a UniPro human protein database (containing 20,387 protein sequences; released on 9 April 2021; http://www.uniprot.org/ (accessed on 6 December 2021)) with PEAKS Studio 7.5 (Bioinformatic Solution, Ontario, CA, USA). The search settings of PEAKS Studio 7.5 combined with UniProt's protein database were as follows: enzyme set to trypsin; up to two missing cut sites; precursor and fragment mass tolerances of 20 ppm and 0.8 Da, respectively; false discovery rate (FDR) of <1%, obtained from a search of the decoy database. Furthermore based on a label-free quantitative analysis, each identified protein had to contain at leas one unique peptide and protein quantification method. Moreover, spectral counts were normalized to the total identification spectrum of each biological sample.

2.5. Enzyme-Linked Immunosorbent Assay (ELISA)

An alpha-2-Heremans–Schmid (HS)-glycoprotein ELISA assay was performed to measure concentrations of AH samples among the single-risk group, double-risk group and the age-matched cataract controls with a Human Alpha-2-HS-glycoprotein ELISA Ki (EH310RB, ThermoFisher Scientific), as per the manufacturer's protocol.

2.6. Statistical Analysis

Clinical data were analyzed using Stata (vers. 16.1, StataCorp, College Station, TX USA) to define the statistical significance between groups by a *t*-test or Chi-squared test and $p < 0.05$ was considered to be statistically significant. Statistical analysis by Fisher's exact test, Wilcoxon test, or Kruskal–Wallis test was used to confirm that there were no statistically significant differences in age among the single-risk group, double-risk group and the age-matched cataract control group (Table 1).

Note: Single risk, patients with the DM or smoking risk factor; double risk, patients with both the DM and smoking risk factors; control, cataract patients with neither of these cataract risk factors; VA, visual acuity; AXL, axial length.

3. Results

Table 1 lists the demographic data of patients with a single risk factor, those with double risk factors, and the control group (with cataract). The mean age of single-risk-factor patients was 72.30 ± 10.14 years, for double-risk-factor patients was 69.38 ± 9.87 years, and for cataract control individuals was 74.00 ± 5.72 years. All patients had cataracts as revealed by a slit lamp examination. The mean protein concentrations were 0.36 ± 0.21 µg/µL in the single-risk-factor group, 0.34 ± 0.11µg/µL in the double-risk-factor group, and 0.22 ± 0.06 µg/µL in the cataract control group. There were statistical differences among total protein contents in these three groups ($p = 0.049$) but no statistical differences in age among these groups ($p = 0.390$). In total, 136 proteins were successfully identified by LC-ESI MS/MS in single-risk-factor, double-risk-factor, and cataract control AH samples (Table 2, Figure 2).

Table 2. List of aqueous humor (AH) proteins identified by LC-ESI-MS/MS.

Q9NQ66	1-phosphatidylinositol 4,5-bisphosphate phosphodiesterase beta-1	P0CG04	Immunoglobulin lambda constant 1
Q99460	26S proteasome non-ATPase regulatory subunit 1	P01700	Immunoglobulin lambda variable 1–47
O95996	Adenomatous polyposis coli protein 2	P0DOX8	Immunoglobulin lambda-1 light chain
P02768	Albumin	B9A064	Immunoglobulin lambda-like polypeptide 5
P51648	Aldehyde dehydrogenase family 3 member A2	P24592	Insulin-like growth factor-binding protein 6
P02763	Alpha-1-acid glycoprotein 1	Q16270	Insulin-like growth factor-binding protein 7
P19652	Alpha-1-acid glycoprotein 2	Q14624	Inter-alpha-trypsin inhibitor heavy chain H4
P01011	Alpha-1-antichymotrypsin	Q6UXX5	Inter-alpha-trypsin inhibitor heavy chain H6
P01009	Alpha-1-antitrypsin	Q17R60	Interphotoreceptor matrix proteoglycan 1
P04217	Alpha-1B-glycoprotein	Q9BZV3	Interphotoreceptor matrix proteoglycan 2
P02765	Alpha-2-HS-glycoprotein	P01042	Kininogen-1
P01023	Alpha-2-macroglobulin	P02750	Leucine-rich alpha-2-glycoprotein
P02489	Alpha-crystallin A chain	Q68G74	LIM/homeobox protein Lhx8
A0A140G945	Alpha-crystallin A2 chain	P51884	Lumican
P02511	Alpha-crystallin B chain	P61626	Lysozyme C
P06733	Alpha-enolase	P01033	Metalloproteinase inhibitor 1
P03950	Angiogenin	P05408	Neuroendocrine protein 7B2
P01019	Angiotensinogen	P61916	NPC intracellular cholesterol transporter 2
P01008	Antithrombin-III	Q9UBM4	Opticin
P02647	Apolipoprotein A-I	P10451	Osteopontin
P02652	Apolipoprotein A-II	Q9UQ90	Paraplegin
P06727	Apolipoprotein A-IV	P36955	Pigment epithelium-derived factor
P05090	Apolipoprotein D	Q15149	Plectin
P02649	Apolipoprotein E	P0CG47	Polyubiquitin-B
P54253	Ataxin-1	P0CG48	Polyubiquitin-C
P02749	Beta-2-glycoprotein 1	Q9ULS6	Potassium voltage-gated channel subfamily S member 2
P61769	Beta-2-microglobulin	O94913	Pre-mRNA cleavage complex 2 protein Pcf11
P05813	Beta-crystallin A3	Q13395	Probable methyltransferase TARBP1
P53674	Beta-crystallin B1	A0A075B6H7	Probable non-functional immunoglobulin kappa variable 3–7
P43320	Beta-crystallin B2	O94823	Probable phospholipid-transporting ATPase VB
P19022	Cadherin-2	Q9UHG2	ProSAAS
P07339	Cathepsin D	P41222	Prostaglandin-H2 D-isomerase
Q8N163	Cell cycle and apoptosis regulator protein 2	Q92520	Protein FAM3C
Q7Z7A1	Centriolin	P05109	Protein S100-A8
P36222	Chitinase-3-like protein 1	Q9H6Z4	Ran-binding protein 3
Q9HAW4	Claspin	P10745	Retinol-binding protein 3
O43809	Cleavage and polyadenylation specificity factor subunit 5	P02753	Retinol-binding protein 4
P10909	Clusterin	P34096	Ribonuclease 4
P01024	Complement C3	P07998	Ribonuclease pancreatic
P0C0L4	Complement C4-A	Q5T481	RNA-binding protein 20

Table 2. *Cont.*

P0C0L5	Complement C4-B	O75326	Semaphorin-7A
P00751	Complement factor B	P02787	Serotransferrin
P00746	Complement factor D	P00441	Superoxide dismutase [Cu-Zn]
P05156	Complement factor I	P05452	Tetranectin
P01034	Cystatin-C	Q8WZ42	Titin
Q8WVS4	Cytoplasmic dynein 2 intermediate chain 1	O15050	TPR and ankyrin repeat-containing protein 1
Q96M86	Dynein heavy chain domain-containing protein 1	Q15582	Transforming growth factor-beta-induced protein ig-h3
P49792	E3 SUMO-protein ligase RanBP2	Q14956	Transmembrane glycoprotein NMB
Q9HC35	Echinoderm microtubule-associated protein-like 4	P02766	Transthyretin
Q13822	Ectonucleotide pyrophosphatase/phosphodiesterase family member 2	P60174	Triosephosphate isomerase
Q8TE68	Epidermal growth factor receptor kinase substrate 8-like protein 1	P35030	Trypsin-3
P02671	Fibrinogen alpha chain	P62979	Ubiquitin-40S ribosomal protein S27a
Q6ZV73	FYVE, RhoGEF and PH domain-containing protein 6	P62987	Ubiquitin-60S ribosomal protein L40
P07320	Gamma-crystallin D	Q5THJ4	Vacuolar protein sorting-associated protein 13D
P22914	Gamma-crystallin S	P02774	Vitamin D-binding protein
P06396	Gelsolin	Q96PQ0	VPS10 domain-containing receptor SorCS2
P22352	Glutathione peroxidase 3	Q9P202	Whirlin
Q14789	Golgin subfamily B member 1	P25311	Zinc-alpha-2-glycoprotein
P00738	Haptoglobin	P0CG04	Immunoglobulin lambda constant 1
P69905	Hemoglobin subunit alpha	P01700	Immunoglobulin lambda variable 1–47
P68871	Hemoglobin subunit beta	P0DOX8	Immunoglobulin lambda-1 light chain
P02042	Hemoglobin subunit delta	B9A064	Immunoglobulin lambda-like polypeptide 5
P02790	Hemopexin	P24592	Insulin-like growth factor-binding protein 6
P62805	Histone H4	Q16270	Insulin-like growth factor-binding protein 7
P0DOX3	Immunoglobulin delta heavy chain	Q14624	Inter-alpha-trypsin inhibitor heavy chain H4
P0DOX5	Immunoglobulin gamma-1 heavy chain	Q6UXX5	Inter-alpha-trypsin inhibitor heavy chain H6
P01859	Immunoglobulin heavy constant gamma 2	Q17R60	Interphotoreceptor matrix proteoglycan 1
P01860	Immunoglobulin heavy constant gamma 3	Q9BZV3	Interphotoreceptor matrix proteoglycan 2
P01861	Immunoglobulin heavy constant gamma 4	P01042	Kininogen-1
P01780	Immunoglobulin heavy variable 3–7	P02750	Leucine-rich alpha-2-glycoprotein
A0A0B4J1Y9	Immunoglobulin heavy variable 3–72	Q68G74	LIM/homeobox protein Lhx8
A0A0B4J1X5	Immunoglobulin heavy variable 3–74	P51884	Lumican
A0A0J9YXX1	Immunoglobulin heavy variable 5-10-1	P61626	Lysozyme C
A0A0B4J1U7	Immunoglobulin heavy variable 6-1	P01033	Metalloproteinase inhibitor 1
P01834	Immunoglobulin kappa constant	P05408	Neuroendocrine protein 7B2
P0DOX7	Immunoglobulin kappa light chain	P61916	NPC intracellular cholesterol transporter 2
P01624	Immunoglobulin kappa variable 3–15	Q9UBM4	Opticin
P01619	Immunoglobulin kappa variable 3–20	P10451	Osteopontin

Comparing the single-risk group to the cataract control group, 125 proteins were found, which included 42 proteins that were present at higher expression levels and 83 proteins that were present at lower expression levels in the single-risk group. In the double-risk group, as compared to the cataract control group, 124 proteins were disclosed, among which 39 proteins had higher expression levels and 85 proteins had lower expression levels in the double-risk group. To understand the biological meaning of the changes of protein expression observed in different risk factor groups, differentially expressed proteins were analyzed for "molecular functions", "biological processes", and "cellular components" by GO annotations. Our results demonstrated that differentially expressed proteins in the three groups had different molecular functions, biological processes, and cellular components (Figure 3). The major biological processes of these proteins were biological regulation, including immune responses, metabolic processes, and responses to stimuli of the AH (Figure 3A). The major molecular functions of AH proteins enriched among single-risk and double-risk patients were antigen binding and enzyme inhibitor activity (Figure 3B). As per cellular component terms of the GO, most significant AH proteins were categorized as extracellular region proteins (Figure 3C). Then, we used Ingenuity Pathway Analysis (IPA, Qiagen) to show canonical pathways that are potentially involved in the pathogenesis of cataracts under the risks of diabetes and smoking. Table 3 lists pathways associated with AH proteins from single-risk patients, double-risk patents, and the cataract controls.

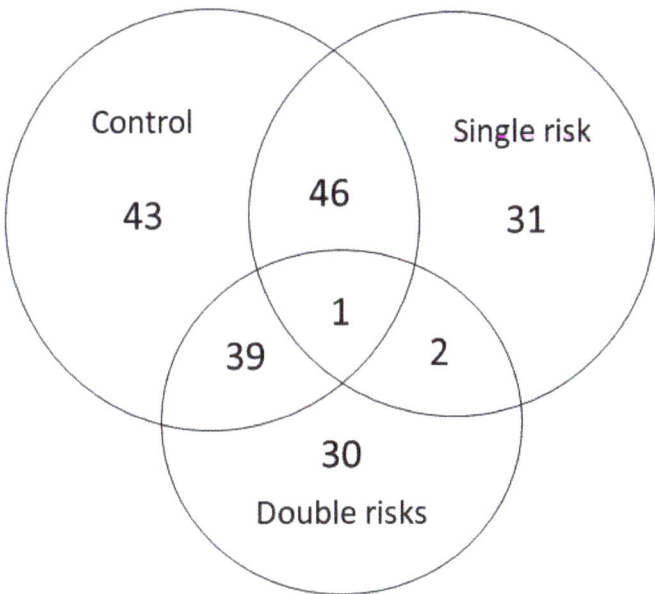

Figure 2. Label-free Nanoflow UHPLC-MS/MS analytical workflow for the proteomic analysis of human aqueous humor. Samples were digested using trypsin and were analyzed using an LTQ-Orbitrap DiscoveryTM hybrid mass spectrometer (Thermo Electron). Proteins were identified and quantified using the SEQUEST algorithm followed by analysis using Xcalibur 2.0 SR1 (Thermo Electron). The intersection of each area represents the number of significant expression ($p < 0.05$) proteins between each groups. Only one protein was significantly deferentially expressed in each group.

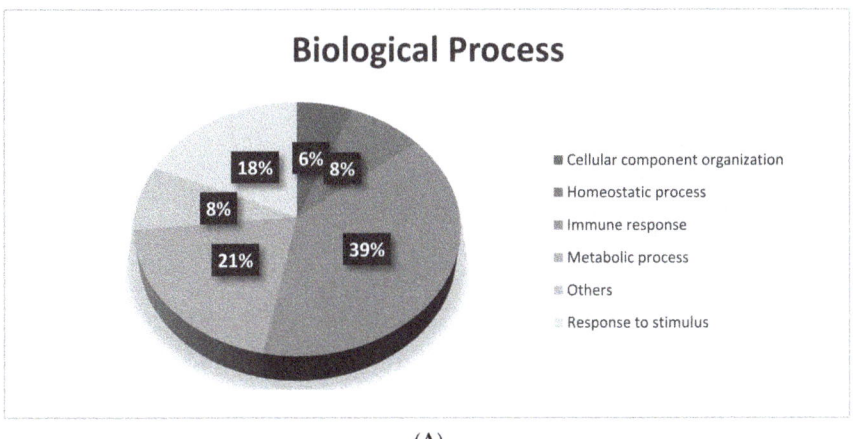

(A)

Figure 3. *Cont.*

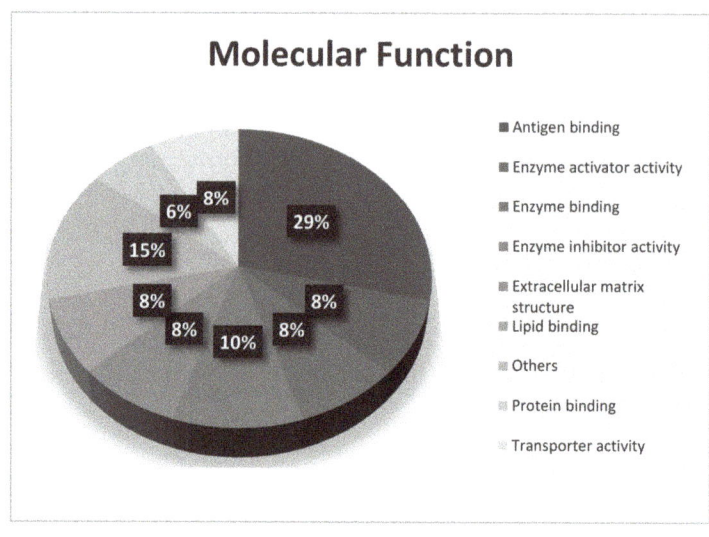

(B)

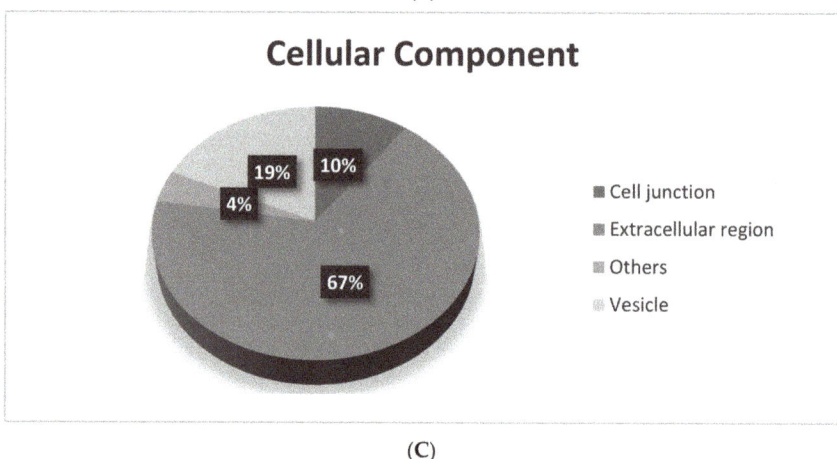

(C)

Figure 3. Gene ontology (GO) analysis of differentially expressed proteins of the aqueous humor (AH) in the cataract control, single-risk, and double-risk groups. We compared identified AH proteins from the three groups: (**A**) biological processes; (**B**) molecular functions; (**C**) cellular components.

The top canonical pathways, including LXR/RXR activation, FXR/RXR activation, and acute-phase response signaling, demonstrated significant associations with AH proteins Statistical analysis was performed on these 136 proteins. In total, 47 proteins exhibited statistically significant changes in content in the group with a single risk factor compared to the cataract control group (Table 4).

Table 3. Pathway analysis of aqueous humor (AH) proteins using IPA tools.

Canonical Pathways	Overlap of Proteins in the Single-Risk and Cataract Control Groups	Overlap of Proteins in the Double-Risk and Cataract Control Groups	Overlap of Proteins in the Single- and Double-Risk Groups
LXR/RXR Activation	12	10	1
FXR/RXR Activation	12	10	1
Acute-Phase Response Signaling	11	11	1
Clathrin-mediated Endocytosis Signaling	12		
Atherosclerosis Signaling	7		
Primary Immunodeficiency Signaling		5	
IL-15 Signaling		9	1
B Cell Receptor Signaling			1

Single risk, patients with the DM or smoking risk factor; double risk, patients with both the DM and smoking risk factors; control, cataract patients with neither of these cataract risk factors.

Table 4. List of selected potential biomarker candidates.

Protein-ID	Protein Name	Cataract Control (Spc)	Single (Spc)	Multiple of Change (Spc)	Cataract Control (Spc)	Double (Spc)	Multiple of Change (Spc)
Q99460	26S proteasome non-ATPase regulatory subunit 1	0.76 ± 1.18	2.99 ± 0.91	3.93	0.76 ± 1.18	2.95 ± 1.90	3.88
P02763	Alpha-1-acid glycoprotein 1	3.26 ± 3.45	0.00 ± 0.00	0	3.26 ± 3.45	0.00 ± 0.00	0
P19652	Alpha-1-acid glycoprotein 2	2.06 ± 1.89	0.00 ± 0.00	0	2.06 ± 1.89	0.00 ± 0.00	0
P01011	Alpha-1-antichymotrypsin	2.87 ± 2.07	0.32 ± 0.52	0.11	2.87 ± 2.07	0.26 ± 0.74	0.09
P02765	Alpha-2-HS-glycoprotein	0.00 ± 0.00	2.14 ± 1.72	−100	0.00 ± 0.00	4.30 ± 2.08	−100
P02647	Apolipoprotein A-I	3.88 ± 4.11	10.49 ± 2.19	2.68	3.88 ± 4.11	9.41 ± 6.49	2.43
P02652	Apolipoprotein A-II	0.09 ± 0.26	2.09 ± 1.33	23.22	0.09 ± 0.26	2.26 ± 1.52	25.11
P02749	Beta-2-glycoprotein 1	1.90 ± 1.49	0.09 ± 0.27	0.05	1.90 ± 1.49	0.33 ± 0.63	0.17
P36222	Chitinase-3-like protein 1	5.39 ± 2.93	1.15 ± 1.87	0.21	5.39 ± 2.93	0.71 ± 0.88	0.13
Q13822	Ectonucleotide pyrophosphatase/phosphodiesterase family member 2	3.63 ± 3.78	0.11 ± 0.34	0.03	3.63 ± 3.78	0.14 ± 0.41	0.04
P22352	Glutathione peroxidase 3	1.15 ± 1.23	0.00 ± 0.00	0	1.15 ± 1.23	0.00 ± 0.00	0
Q14789	Golgin subfamily B member 1	0.54 ± 0.71	0.00 ± 0.00	0	0.54 ± 0.71	0.00 ± 0.00	0
P02790	Hemopexin	21.12 ± 8.44	1.56 ± 1.62	0.07	21.12 ± 8.44	2.67 ± 3.40	0.13
P0DOX5	Immunoglobulin gamma-1 heavy chain	34.76 ± 6.08	10.24 ± 4.37	0.29	34.76 ± 6.08	10.58 ± 5.89	0.3
P01859	Immunoglobulin heavy constant gamma 2	21.29 ± 3.52	5.29 ± 3.57	0.25	21.29 ± 3.52	6.27 ± 4.97	0.3
P01860	Immunoglobulin heavy constant gamma 3	22.01 ± 4.99	6.75 ± 3.30	0.31	22.01 ± 4.99	6.98 ± 4.25	0.32
P01861	Immunoglobulin heavy constant gamma 4	15.02 ± 3.42	4.14 ± 2.88	0.28	15.02 ± 3.42	4.92 ± 2.49	0.33
P01780	Immunoglobulin heavy variable 3-7	2.46 ± 2.13	0.00 ± 0.00	0	2.46 ± 2.13	0.25 ± 0.72	0.1
A0A0B4J1Y9	Immunoglobulin heavy variable 3-72	1.67 ± 1.09	0.00 ± 0.00	0	1.67 ± 1.09	0.13 ± 0.36	0.08
A0A0B4J1X5	Immunoglobulin heavy variable 3-74	2.08 ± 1.99	0.00 ± 0.00	0	2.08 ± 1.99	0.25 ± 0.72	0.12
A0A0B4J1U7	Immunoglobulin heavy variable 6-1	1.16 ± 1.28	0.09 ± 0.27	0.08	1.16 ± 1.28	0.00 ± 0.00	0
P01834	Immunoglobulin kappa constant	16.50 ± 5.02	2.75 ± 2.24	0.17	16.50 ± 5.02	2.94 ± 2.81	0.18
P0DOX7	Immunoglobulin kappa light chain	12.23 ± 3.03	2.75 ± 2.24	0.23	12.23 ± 3.03	2.94 ± 2.81	0.24
P0CG01	Immunoglobulin lambda constant 1	4.74 ± 1.71	2.29 ± 1.75	0.48	4.74 ± 1.71	1.66 ± 1.20	0.35
P0DOX8	Immunoglobulin lambda-1 light chain	4.74 ± 1.71	2.29 ± 1.75	0.48	4.74 ± 1.71	1.66 ± 1.20	0.35

Table 4. Cont.

Protein-ID	Protein Name	Cataract Control (Spc)	Single (Spc)	Multiple of Change (Spc)	Cataract Control (Spc)	Double (Spc)	Multiple of Change (Spc)
B9A064	Immunoglobulin lambda-like polypeptide 5	4.74 ± 1.71	2.29 ± 1.75	0.48	4.74 ± 1.71	1.66 ± 1.20	0.35
Q16270	Insulin-like growth factor-binding protein 7	3.52 ± 1.34	1.83 ± 1.03	0.52	3.52 ± 1.34	1.09 ± 1.28	0.31
P01033	Metalloproteinase inhibitor 1	0.78 ± 0.80	0.00 ± 0.00	0	0.78 ± 0.80	0.00 ± 0.00	0
P61916	NPC intracellular cholesterol transporter 2	1.05 ± 0.89	0.00 ± 0.00	0	1.05 ± 0.89	0.20 ± 0.58	0.19
Q92520	Protein FAM3C	1.50 ± 1.23	0.00 ± 0.00	0	1.50 ± 1.23	0.00 ± 0.00	0
P02753	Retinol-binding protein 4	2.09 ± 0.97	0.71 ± 1.30	0.34	2.09 ± 0.97	0.86 ± 0.96	0.41
O75326	Semaphorin-7A	0.98 ± 1.59	0.00 ± 0.00	0	0.98 ± 1.59	0.00 ± 0.00	0
P02787	Serotransferrin	74.79 ± 23.85	31.40 ± 9.50	0.42	74.79 ± 23.85	30.22 ± 9.85	0.4
P00441	Superoxide dismutase [Cu-Zn]	2.93 ± 1.87	0.19 ± 0.41	0.06	2.93 ± 1.87	0.25 ± 0.72	0.09
P05452	Tetranectin	2.53 ± 1.41	0.00 ± 0.00	0	2.53 ± 1.41	0.00 ± 0.00	0
P25311	Zinc-alpha-2-glycoprotein	8.92 ± 2.57	0.00 ± 0.00	0	8.92 ± 2.57	0.52 ± 1.12	0.06
P06727	Apolipoprotein A-IV	0.11 ± 0.32	5.51 ± 4.11	50.09			
P02649	Apolipoprotein E	1.04 ± 1.80	3.92 ± 2.74	3.77			
O43809	Cleavage and polyadenylation specificity factor subunit 5	0.98 ± 0.68	0.21 ± 0.68	0.21			
P01619	Immunoglobulin kappa variable 3-20	1.06 ± 1.34	0.00 ± 0.00	0			
P24592	Insulin-like growth factor-binding protein 6	1.88 ± 1.31	0.23 ± 0.72	0.12			
Q9UBM4	Opticin	0.09 ± 0.26	0.64 ± 0.74	7.11			
P0CG47	Polyubiquitin-B	1.54 ± 1.41	0.10 ± 0.33	0.06			
P0CG48	Polyubiquitin-C	1.54 ± 1.41	0.10 ± 0.33	0.06			
Q9ULS6	Potassium voltage-gated channel subfamily S member 2	0.11 ± 0.32	0.65 ± 0.75	5.91			
P62979	Ubiquitin-40S ribosomal protein S27a	1.54 ± 1.41	0.10 ± 0.33	0.06			
P62987	Ubiquitin-60S ribosomal protein L40	1.54 ± 1.41	0.10 ± 0.33	0.06			
P61769	Beta-2-microglobulin				5.22 ± 2.45	2.02 ± 1.83	0.39
P0COL4	Complement C4-A				0.41 ± 0.82	2.16 ± 2.53	5.27
P0COL5	Complement C4-B				0.41 ± 0.82	2.16 ± 2.53	5.27
P41222	Prostaglandin-H2 D-isomerase				11.39 ± 1.97	8.00 ± 1.65	0.71

Single risk, patients with the DM or smoking risk factor; double risk, patients with both the DM and smoking risk factors; control, cataract patients with neither of these cataract risk factors; Spc, spectral count.

In a comparison of the double-risk-factor group with the cataract control group, 40 proteins were statistically significantly ($p < 0.05$) expressed (Table 4). Among the 51 proteins that were significantly changed, 10 proteins were increased in the single- or double-risk groups, including 26S proteasome non-ATPase regulatory subunit 1, alpha-2-HS-glycoprotein, apolipoprotein A-I, apolipoprotein A-II, apolipoprotein A-IV, apolipoprotein E, opticin, potassium voltage-gated channel subfamily S member 2, complement C4-A, and complement C4-B. Another 41 proteins exhibited decreased expression in the single- or double-risk groups compared to cataract controls (Table 4). In particular, alpha-2-HS-glycoprotein was the only one that presented a significant change among all three of the groups (cataract control vs. single: $p = 0.00338$; cataract control vs. double: $p = 0.00062$; single vs. double: $p = 0.03309$), which demonstrated an increasing trend with increase in risk (Figure 4).

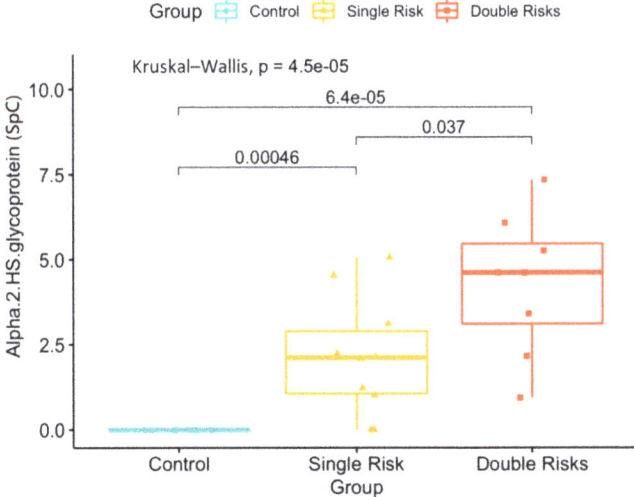

Figure 4. Proteomics analysis revealed significant concentration changes in the alpha-2-HS-glycoprotein (SpC, spectral count) among the three groups. Single risk, patients with the diabetes mellitus (DM) or smoking risk factor; double risk, patients with both the DM and smoking risk factors; control, cataract patients with neither of these cataract risk factors.

Furthermore, we performed an ELISA analysis to determine the concentration of alpha-2-HS-glycoprotein. Compared to the cataract control group, the average concentration of alpha-2-HS-glycoprotein was significantly higher in single-risk-factor group (0.43 µg/mL) patients (0.16 µg/mL) ($p = 0.002$) (Figure 5).

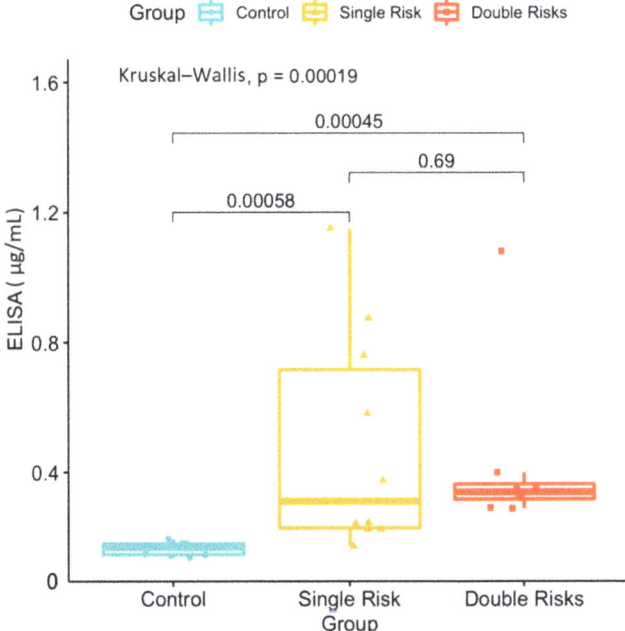

Figure 5. ELISA analysis of significant concentration (µg/mL) changes of the alpha-2-HS-glycoprotein

between risk factor and cataract control groups. However, there was no significant concentration change between the single- and double-risk-factor groups. Single risk, patients with the diabetes mellitus (DM) or smoking risk factor; double risk, patients with both the DM and smoking risk factors; control, cataract patients with neither of these cataract risk factors.

Furthermore, the average concentration significantly increased in double-risk-factor group (0.43 µg/mL) patients compared to the cataract control group (0.16 µg/mL) ($p < 0.001$) (Figure 5). The ELISA analysis revealed significant concentration changes between the risk factor and cataract control groups. However, there was no significant concentration change between the single- and double-risk-factor groups. A subgroup analysis was performed to confirm that DM and smoking risk factors significantly influenced the ELISA concentration compared to the cataract control group (Figure 6).

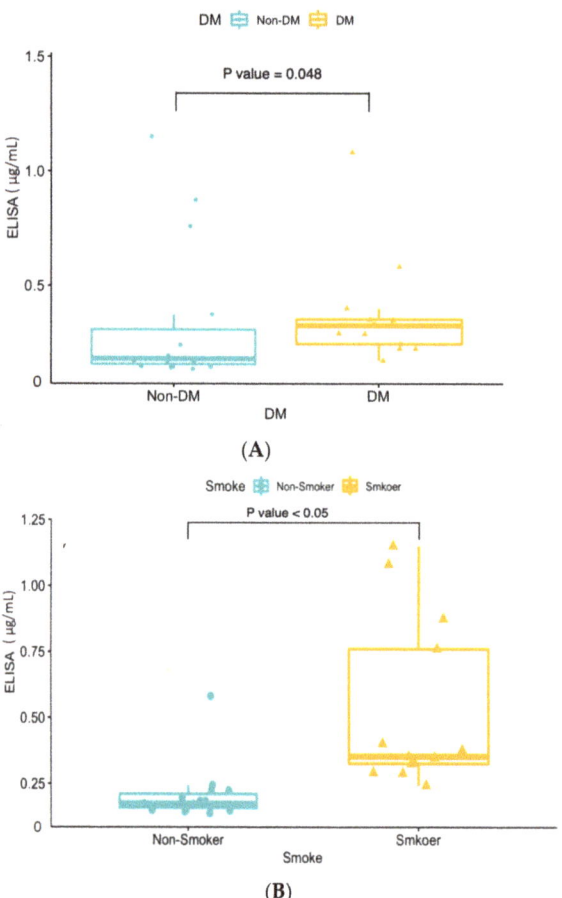

Figure 6. (A) ELISA analysis of significant concentration (µg/mL) changes in the alpha-2-HS glycoprotein between the diabetes mellitus (DM) groups and cataract control group. (B) ELISA analysis of significant concentration (µg/mL) changes in the alpha-2-HS-glycoprotein between the smoking groups and cataract control group. DM group ($n = 13$): DM single-risk patients ($n = 5$) + double-risk patients ($n = 8$); Non-DM group ($n = 14$): smoking single-risk patients ($n = 5$) + cataract control group ($n = 9$); Smokers ($n = 13$): smoking single-risk patients ($n = 5$) + double-risk patients ($n = 8$); Non-smokers ($n = 14$): DM single-risk patients ($n = 5$) + cataract control group ($n = 9$).

In our study, we analyzed the aqueous protein contents of the AH samples of single-risk and double-risk patients and a control group (with cataract) using label-free n-UPLC-MS/MS quantitation. We reported that in cataract patients with different risk profiles, 51 AH proteins were significantly changed compared to cataract controls. The alpha-2-HS-glycoprotein was significantly differently expressed between risk groups and cataract controls and could be a potential aqueous protein marker for detecting smoking and DM cataract risk factors. The increased levels of total protein concentrations were reported in the AH, which provides a possible marker to monitor the AH of cataract risk exposure. Note that additional studies exploring the roles of this protein in the development or the pathogenesis molecular pathway of cataracts would be beneficial. To our knowledge, this is the first study to analyze how cataract risk factors influenced the AH in the development of cataract disease. We reported that only one protein had significantly changed, which was the alpha-2-HS-glycoprotein; its expression increased in the presence of risk factors. Alpha-2-HS-glycoprotein, known as fetuin-A, was reported to be a systemic inhibitor of precipitation of basic calcium phosphate, thereby preventing unwanted calcification [15] and influencing the mineral phase of bone [16]. The alpha-2-HS-glycoprotein is synthesized in the liver, electively concentrated in the bone matrix, and secreted in plasma. The dysfunction of the gene represented by this entry is associated with alopecia-mental retardation syndrome [17]. There was previous evidence demonstrating that the alpha-2-HS-glycoprotein was present in the rabbit AH following two different cataract surgery incision procedures [18]; furthermore, there were significant decreases in the AH of 5-year-old buphthalmic rabbits [19] but not in the 2-year-old group, demonstrating that alpha-2-HS-glycoprotein alters with pathologic changes in DM, anterior lens capsule, and the angular meshwork. In humans, it was shown to be an inhibitor of transforming growth factor (TGF)-β2 [20], a protein that shows increased expression in the trabecular meshwork (TM) in open-angle glaucoma causing extracellular matrix (ECM) deposition in the human TM [21]. The alpha-2-HS-glycoprotein inhibits bone morphogenetic proteins that are changed in the TM in open-angle glaucoma [22]. This evidence suggests the potential interactions of the alpha-2-HS-glycoprotein with multiple proteins that are important in open-angle glaucoma. However, there is scarce evidence demonstrating a relationship between the alpha-2-HS-glycoprotein and cataract disease in human beings to date. Interestingly, the serum levels of alpha-2-HS-glycoprotein, called fetuin-A, are known to be highly associated with DM in humans. Initially, it was discussed in the context of preventing glucose toxicity in early 2002 [23,24]. Then, in the past two decades, the alpha-2-HS-glycoprotein was linked to insulin resistance, obesity, and cardiovascular diseases [25–31]. Guo et al. and Roshanzamir et al. revealed evidence using meta-analyses that higher serum alpha-2-HS-glycoprotein levels are associated with increased risk of type 2 DM [32,33]. All these previous studies reported the correlation of alpha-2-HS-glycoprotein levels in urine [34] or serum [35] with diabetes. Yuksel et al. performed a serum and AH alpha-2-HS-glycoprotein (fetuin-A) level comparison in pseudoexfoliation syndrome (PEXS) patients [36]. They found significantly increased alpha-2-HS-glycoprotein levels in the AH of patients with PEXS, but no correlation between the AH and serum levels of alpha-2-HS-glycoprotein between the groups. They suggested that the increase in alpha-2-HS-glycoprotein levels in the AH was due to disruption of the blood–aqueous barrier because of the hypoperfusion and anterior chamber hypoxia in PEXS. Thus, until now there was scarce evidence to prove that the serum level of alpha-2-HS-glycoprotein was associated with that in AH. However, our results are the first to report that human aqueous levels of the alpha-2-HS-glycoprotein are associated with diabetes risk factors for cataract formation. The ELISA confirmation of aqueous alpha-2-HS-glycoprotein levels confirmed these results. In certain diabetic patients, we provide a novel way of thinking about changes in alpha-2-HS-glycoprotein levels in the circulation and in the aqueous fluid. We suggest that the alpha-2-HS-glycoprotein could be an aqueous-specific marker of cataract risk, which is highly associated with diabetes. The alpha-2-HS-glycoprotein is known as an immune-reactive protein that was determined to be smoking- and age-associated with the development of head and neck cancers. The consistent association of chronic smoking shows an immune reactivity status that changes the serum levels of alpha-2-HS-glycoprotein in head and neck cancer patients [37]. Marechal et al. demonstrated a negative correlation between serum fetuin-A levels and a history of smoking, in which fetuin-A levels were determined by a common haplotype of the *AHSG* gene, low plasma cholesterol, and a history of smoking in renal transplant recipients [38]. They considered that it might reflect consequences of tobacco smoking on liver function, physical activity, or weight loss, which increased aortic calcification and risk of cardiovascular events in renal transplant recipients. These previous studies support our result that the alpha-2-HS-glycoprotein may be associated with the smoking habit. We considered that the alpha-2-HS-glycoprotein could be an aqueous-specific marker of cataract risks that is highly associated with smoking However, multiple limitations of this study should be reported. First, only eight to ten samples in each group were investigated, and future large-scale studies could help confirm our results. The small sample numbers may be attributed to ELISA, which could not validate the proportional results of aqueous alpha-2-HS-glycoprotein levels in the three groups. Second, only a small amount of AH could be obtained because of anatomical features, which limited our ability to conduct subsequent validation assays. Third, the development of multiplex immunoassays can be improved. Finally, we can only provide the results of proteomic and ELISA data correlated with smoking and DM risk factors. The exact pathway by which the alpha-2-HS-glycoprotein is involved in cataract pathogenesis remains unclear. More future investigations of molecular pathways are required to discuss how and why the proteomics data varied with smoking and DM, and finally to supply better knowledge of cataracts for the whole of humanity. More studies are also required to analyze the alpha-2-HS-glycoprotein levels in AH of non-diabetic cataract patients, along with further serum and AH comparison analyses of cataract patients with diabetes. In conclusion, our results are from a pioneering exploration of the protein profile for the risk factors involved in cataracts. Cataracts form because of a complicated pathological process involving several proteins that participate in immune reactions and metabolic processes that were identified in AH using a proteomics analysis. The alpha-2-HS-glycoprotein, called fetuin-a, could be a potential aqueous biomarker associated with DM and smoking, which are cataract risk factors. Additional studies are required to complete the analysis and to understand the functions of these cataract-specific proteins, which could provide significant information for the diagnosis, clinical treatment, and prognosis of cataracts.

Author Contributions: Conceptualization, W.-C.C. and C.-W.C.; methodology, C.-C.L. and C.-W.C.; software, C.-C.L. and C.-H.L.; validation, W.-C.C., C.-W.C. and S.-H.C.; formal analysis, C.-H.L.; investigation, W.-C.C.; writing—original draft preparation, W.-C.C.; writing—review and editing, C.-W.C.; visualization, C.-C.L.; supervision, C.-W.C.; funding acquisition, W.-C.C. All authors have read and agreed to the published version of the manuscript.

Funding: This research received no external funding.

Institutional Review Board Statement: The study was conducted according to the guidelines of the Declaration of Helsinki, and approved by the Institutional Review Board of Taoyuan General Hospital, Ministry of Health and Welfare (TYGH109009 and 30 April 2020) (Taoyuan, Taiwan).

Informed Consent Statement: Informed consent was obtained from all subjects involved in the study. Written informed consent has been obtained from the patients to publish this paper.

Data Availability Statement: Not applicable.

Conflicts of Interest: The authors declare no conflict of interest. The funders had no role in the design of the study; in the collection, analyses, or interpretation of data; in the writing of the manuscript, or in the decision to publish the results.

References

1. Rao, G.N.; Khanna, R.; Payal, A. The global burden of cataract. *Curr. Opin. Ophthalmol.* **2011**, *22*, 4–9. [CrossRef] [PubMed]
2. Liu, Y.C.; Wilkins, M.; Kim, T.; Malyugin, B.; Mehta, J.S. Cataracts. *Lancet* **2017**, *390*, 600–612. [CrossRef]

1. Pascolini, D.; Mariotti, S.P. Global estimates of visual impairment: 2010. *Br. J. Ophthalmol.* **2012**, *96*, 614–618. [CrossRef] [PubMed]
2. Mukesh, B.N.; Le, A.; Dimitrov, P.N.; Ahmed, S.; Taylor, H.R.; McCarty, C.A. Development of cataract and associated risk factors: The Visual Impairment Project. *Arch. Ophthalmol.* **2006**, *124*, 79–85. [CrossRef] [PubMed]
3. Foster, P.J.; Wong, T.Y.; Machin, D.; Johnson, G.J.; Seah, S.K.L. Risk factors for nuclear, cortical and posterior subcapsular cataracts in the Chinese population of Singapore: The Tanjong Pagar Survey. *Br. J. Ophthalmol.* **2003**, *87*, 1112–1120. [CrossRef]
4. Becker, C.; Schneider, C.; Aballéa, S.; Bailey, C.; Bourne, R.; Jick, S.; Meier, C. Cataract in patients with diabetes mellitus-incidence rates in the UK and risk factors. *Eye* **2018**, *32*, 1028–1035. [CrossRef] [PubMed]
5. Pan, C.W.; Boey, P.Y.; Cheng, C.Y.; Saw, S.M.; Tay, W.T.; Wang, J.J.; Tan, A.G.; Mitchell, P.; Wong, T.Y. Myopia, axial length, and age-related cataract: The Singapore Malay eye study. *Investig. Ophthalmol. Vis. Sci.* **2013**, *54*, 4498–4502. [CrossRef]
6. Kyselova, Z. Mass spectrometry-based proteomics approaches applied in cataract research. *Mass. Spectrom. Rev.* **2011**, *30*, 1173–1184. [CrossRef]
7. Truscott, R.J.; Friedrich, M.G. Old proteins and the Achilles heel of mass spectrometry. The role of proteomics in the etiology of human cataract. *Proteom. Clin. Appl.* **2014**, *8*, 195–203. [CrossRef]
8. Zhang, B.N.; Wu, X.; Dai, Y.; Qi, B.; Fan, C.; Huang, Y. Proteomic analysis of aqueous humor from cataract patients with retinitis pigmentosa. *J. Cell. Physiol.* **2021**, *236*, 2659–2668. [CrossRef]
9. Bennett, K.L.; Funk, M.; Tschernutter, M.; Breitwieser, F.P.; Planyavsky, M.; Mohien, C.U.; Müller, A.; Trajanoski, Z.; Colinge, J.; Giulio, S.F.; et al. Proteomic analysis of human cataract aqueous humour: Comparison of one-dimensional gel LCMS with two-dimensional LCMS of unlabelled and iTRAQ(R)-labelled specimens. *J. Proteom.* **2011**, *74*, 151–166. [CrossRef] [PubMed]
10. Schey, K.L.; Wang, Z.; Friedrich, M.G.; Garland, D.L.; Truscott, R.J.W. Spatiotemporal changes in the human lens proteome: Critical insights into long-lived proteins. *Prog. Retin. Eye Res.* **2020**, *76*, 1008–1902. [CrossRef] [PubMed]
11. Ji, Y.; Rong, X.; Ye, H.; Zhang, K.; Lu, Y. Proteomic analysis of aqueous humor proteins associated with cataract development. *Clin. Biochem.* **2015**, *48*, 1304–1309. [CrossRef] [PubMed]
12. Kim, T.W.; Kang, J.W.; Ahn, J.; Lee, E.K.; Cho, K.C.; Han, B.N.R.; Hong, N.Y.; Park, J.; Kim, K.P. Proteomic analysis of the aqueous humor in age-related macular degeneration (AMD) patients. *J. Proteome Res.* **2012**, *11*, 4034–4043. [CrossRef]
13. Heiss, A.; Chesne, A.D.; Denecke, B.; Grötzinger, J.; Yamamoto, K.; Renné, T.; Dechent, W.J. Structural basis of calcification inhibition by alpha 2-HS glycoprotein/fetuin-A. Formation of colloidal calciprotein particles. *J. Biol. Chem.* **2003**, *278*, 1333–1341. [CrossRef] [PubMed]
14. Lee, C.C.; Bowman, B.H.; Yang, F.M. Human alpha 2-HS-glycoprotein: The A and B chains with a connecting sequence are encoded by a single mRNA transcript. *Proc. Natl. Acad. Sci. USA* **1987**, *84*, 4403–4407. [CrossRef]
15. Reza Sailani, M.; Jahanbani, F.; Nasiri, J.; Behnam, M.; Salehi, M.; Sedghi, M.; Hoseinzadeh, M.; Takahashi, S.; Zia, A.; Gruber, J.; et al. Association of AHSG with alopecia and mental retardation (APMR) syndrome. *Hum. Genet.* **2017**, *136*, 287–296. [CrossRef] [PubMed]
16. Stastna, M.; Behrens, A.; McDonnell, P.J.; Jennifer, E.V.E. Analysis of protein composition of rabbit aqueous humor following two different cataract surgery incision procedures using 2-DE and LC-MS/MS. *Proteome Sci.* **2011**, *9*, 8. [CrossRef]
17. Edward, D.P.; Bouhenni, R. Anterior segment alterations and comparative aqueous humor proteomics in the buphthalmic rabbit (an American Ophthalmological Society thesis). *Trans. Am. Ophthalmol. Soc.* **2011**, *109*, 66–114.
18. Szweras, M.; Liu, D.; Partridge, E.A.; Pawling, J.; Sukhu, B.; Clokie, C.; Dechent, W.J.; Tenenbaum, H.C.; Swallow, C.J.; Grynpas, M.D.; et al. Alpha 2-HS glycoprotein/fetuin, a transforming growth factor-beta/bone morphogenetic protein antagonist, regulates postnatal bone growth and remodeling. *J. Biol. Chem.* **2002**, *277*, 19991–19997. [CrossRef]
19. Wordinger, R.J.; Fleenor, D.L.; Hellberg, P.E.; Pang, I.H.; Tovar, T.O.; Zode, G.S.; Fuller, J.A.; Clark, A.F. Effects of TGF-beta2, BMP-4, and gremlin in the trabecular meshwork: Implications for glaucoma. *Investig. Ophthalmol. Vis. Sci.* **2007**, *48*, 1191–1200. [CrossRef] [PubMed]
20. Umulis, D.; O'Connor, M.B.; Blair, S.S. The extracellular regulation of bone morphogenetic protein signaling. *Development* **2009**, *136*, 3715–3728. [CrossRef] [PubMed]
21. Arnaud, P.; Kalabay, L. Alpha2-HS glycoprotein: A protein in search of a function. *Diabetes Metab. Res. Rev.* **2002**, *18*, 311–314. [CrossRef] [PubMed]
22. Ren, J.; Davidoff, A.J. Alpha2-Heremans Schmid glycoprotein, a putative inhibitor of tyrosine kinase, prevents glucose toxicity associated with cardiomyocyte dysfunction. *Diabetes Metab. Res. Rev.* **2002**, *18*, 305–310. [CrossRef]
23. Trepanowski, J.F.; Mey, J.; Varady, K.A. Fetuin-A: A novel link between obesity and related complications. *Int. J. Obes.* **2015**, *39*, 734–741. [CrossRef]
24. Jung, T.W.; Yoo, H.J.; Choi, K.M. Implication of hepatokines in metabolic disorders and cardiovascular diseases. *BBA Clin.* **2016**, *5*, 108–113. [CrossRef]
25. Dabrowska, A.M.; Stanislaw Tarach, J.S.; Duma, B.W.; Duma, D. Fetuin-A (AHSG) and its usefulness in clinical practice. Review of the literature. *Biomed. Pap. Med. Fac. Univ. Palacky Olomouc Czech Repub.* **2015**, *159*, 352–359. [CrossRef] [PubMed]
26. Singh, M.; Sharma, P.K.; Garg, V.K.; Mondal, S.C.; Singh, A.K.; Kumar, N. Role of fetuin-A in atherosclerosis associated with diabetic patients. *J. Pharm. Pharmacol.* **2012**, *64*, 1703–1708. [CrossRef]
27. Rasul, S.; Wagner, L.; Kautzky-Willer, A. Fetuin-A and angiopoietins in obesity and type 2 diabetes mellitus. *Endocrine* **2012**, *42*, 496–505. [CrossRef]
28. Mori, K.; Emoto, M.; Inaba, M. Fetuin-A and the cardiovascular system. *Adv. Clin. Chem.* **2012**, *56*, 175–195. [PubMed]

31. Horshuns'ka, M.; Karachentsev, I.L.; Kravchun, N.O.; Iensen, E.; Leshchenko, Z.A.; Hladkykh, O.I.; Krasova, N.S.; Tyzhnenko, T.V.; Opaleĭko, I.A.; Poltorak, V.V. Biological role of fetuin A and its potential importance for prediction of cardiovascular risk in patients with type 2 diabetes mellitus. *Ukr. Biokhim. Zh.* **2013**, *85*, 10–21.
32. Guo, V.Y.; Cao, B.; Cai, C.; Cheng, K.K.Y.; Cheung, B.M.Y. Fetuin-A levels and risk of type 2 diabetes mellitus: A systematic review and meta-analysis. *Acta Diabetol.* **2018**, *55*, 87–98. [CrossRef] [PubMed]
33. Roshanzamir, F.; Miraghajani, M.; Rouhani, M.H.; Mansourian, M.; Ghiasvand, R.; Safavi, S.M. The association between circulating fetuin-A levels and type 2 diabetes mellitus risk: Systematic review and meta-analysis of observational studies. *J. Endocrinol. Investig.* **2018**, *41*, 33–47. [CrossRef] [PubMed]
34. Inoue, K.; Wada, J.; Eguchi, J.; Nakatsuka, A.; Teshigawara, S.; Murakami, K.; Ogawa, D.; Takahiro, T. Urinary fetuin-A is a novel marker for diabetic nephropathy in type 2 diabetes identified by lectin microarray. *PLoS ONE* **2013**, *8*, e77118. [CrossRef]
35. Ou, H.Y.; Yang, Y.C.; Wu, H.T.; Wu, J.S.; Lu, F.H.; Chang, C.J. Serum fetuin-A concentrations are elevated in subjects with impaired glucose tolerance and newly diagnosed type 2 diabetes. *Clin. Endocrinol.* **2011**, *75*, 450–455. [CrossRef] [PubMed]
36. Yuksel, N.; Takmaz, T.; Turkcu, U.O.; Ergin, M.; Altinkaynak, H.; Bilgihan, A. Serum and Aqueous Humor Levels of Fetuin-A in Pseudoexfoliation Syndrome. *Curr. Eye Res.* **2017**, *42*, 1378–1381. [CrossRef]
37. Wolf, G.T.; Chretien, P.B.; Weiss, J.F.; Edwards, B.K.; Spiegel, H.E. Effects of smoking and age on serum levels of immune reactive proteins. *Otolaryngol. Head Neck Surg.* **1982**, *90*, 319–326.
38. Marechal, C.; Schlieper, G.; Nguyen, P.; Krüger, T.; Coche, E.; Robert, A.; Floege, J.; Goffin, E.; Jadoul, M.; Devuyst, O. Serum fetuin-A levels are associated with vascular calcifications and predict cardiovascular events in renal transplant recipients. *Clin. J. Am. Soc. Nephrol.* **2011**, *6*, 974–985. [CrossRef]

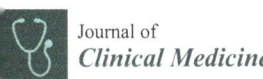

Article

Development of a New Method for Calculating Intraocular Lens Power after Myopic Laser In Situ Keratomileusis by Combining the Anterior–Posterior Ratio of the Corneal Radius of the Curvature with the Double-K Method

Yoshihiko Iida [1,*], Kimiya Shimizu [2] and Nobuyuki Shoji [1]

1. Department of Ophthalmology, Kitasato University School of Medicine, Sagamihara 252-0374, Japan; nshoji@kitasato-u.ac.jp
2. Eye Center, Sanno Hospital, Tokyo 107-0052, Japan; kimiyas@iuhw.ac.jp
* Correspondence: yiida@kitasato-u.ac.jp

Abstract: Background: A new method, the Iida–Shimizu–Shoji (ISS) method, is proposed for calculating intraocular lens (IOL) power that combines the anterior–posterior ratio of the corneal radius of the curvature after laser in situ keratomileusis (LASIK) and to compare the predictability of the method with that of other IOL formulas after LASIK. Methods: The estimated corneal power before LASIK (Kpre) in the double-K method was 43.86 D according to the American Society of Cataract and Refractive Surgery calculator, and the K readings of the IOL master were used as the K values after LASIK (Kpost). The factor for correcting the target refractive value (correcting factor [C-factor]) was calculated from the correlation between the anterior–posterior ratio of the corneal radius of the curvature and the refractive error obtained using this method for 30 eyes of 30 patients. Results: Fifty-nine eyes of 59 patients were included. The mean values of the numerical and absolute prediction errors obtained using the ISS method were −0.02 ± 0.45 diopter (D) and 0.35 ± 0.27 D, respectively. The prediction errors using the ISS method were within ±0.25, ±0.50, and ±1.00 D in 49.2%, 76.3%, and 96.6% of the eyes, respectively. The predictability of the ISS method was comparable to or better than some of the other formulas. Conclusions: The ISS method is useful for calculating the IOL power in eyes treated with cataract surgery after LASIK.

Keywords: IOL power calculation after LASIK; no-history method; cataract surgery; anterior–posterior ratio of the corneal radius of the curvature

1. Introduction

The opportunities to perform cataract surgery in patients who have undergone corneal refractive surgeries such as laser in situ keratomileusis (LASIK) are increasing. The problem in performing cataract surgery after corneal refractive surgery is the incorrect IOL power calculation. Especially, the result of the IOL power calculation after myopic corneal refractive surgery causes a hyperopic shift [1–5]. The reason for residual hyperopia is inaccurate measurement of K value after corneal refractive surgery and incorrect effective lens position (ELP) calculated using third-generation theoretical formulas in which the post-corneal refractive surgery K value that was flattened is used [6,7]. A number of theoretical and empirical approaches have been proposed to solve this problem [1–5,7–27].

Among the approaches, the double-K method, described by Arramberri [7] in 2003, enables more accurate IOL power calculation by estimating the ELP using pre-refractive surgery corneal measurements (Kpre) and the subjective refractive value-derived K values (clinical history method) as Kpost for optical calculations without using the post-refractive surgery corneal measurements. This principle makes sense; however, many patients unfortunately do not have the necessary data for the clinical history method, such as Kpre and subjective refractive values before and after refractive surgery.

Corneal refractive power measurements are inaccurate in the post-refractive surgery eye, because the assumption of estimating total corneal refractive power from the radius of the curvature of the corneal anterior surface, an algorithm used by keratometers and topographers, is not valid. The reason is the change in the relationship between the anterior and posterior corneal radii of the curvature, which is no longer 7.5/6.3 [8]. This invalidates the value of the different corneal indexes of refraction (standardized index of refraction = 1.3375), which allows total corneal power calculation from the anterior surface radius of the curvature in nonoperated eyes [9,10]. The Scheimpflug anterior segment imaging system (Pentacam, Oculus GmbH) can measure the posterior corneal radii. Excimer laser ablation thins the corneal thickness and flattens the curvature plane of the anterior cornea, which changes the corneal refractive power. In the case of excimer laser ablation, the greater the amount of correction and anterior–posterior ratio of the corneal radius, the greater the error in the K value.

In cases where the double-K method is performed (in which we do not have pre-refractive surgery data), the prediction error is expected to depend on the anterior–posterior ratio of the corneal radius when using postoperative keratometric K values for the double-K method. This study devised a new no-history method, the Iida–Shimizu–Shoji (ISS) method, based on the double-K method using the prediction error induced by the ratio of the anterior and posterior radii of the corneal curvature after LASIK. This method can calculate IOL frequencies without relying on preoperative data. The accuracy of this new method was compared with other formulas in eyes after LASIK.

2. Materials and Methods

2.1. Patients and Methods

This study included Japanese patients who underwent cataract surgery after LASIK at the Department of Ophthalmology, Kitasato University Hospital. This retrospective review of the data was approved by the Institutional Review Board at the Kitasato University (B17-292) and conformed to the Declaration of Helsinki.

2.2. Cataract Surgical Procedures

For the cataract surgery, standard phacoemulsification was performed using topical anesthesia. The surgical technique consisted of capsulorhexis, nucleus, and cortex extractions, as well as IOL implantation, through a 2.8 mm temporal clear corneal incision, in all the cases. Nontoric monofocal IOLs (AQ-110NV, STAAR Surgical, Chiba, Japan) were implanted. All the surgeries were uneventfully performed by two experienced surgeons (Y.I. and K.S.) using the same technique.

2.3. Estimation of Refractive Error in the Double-K Method Induced by the Anterior–Posterior Ratio of the Corneal Radii

To establish a method for estimating the refractive error in the double-K method induced by the anterior–posterior ratio of the corneal radii, we retrospectively studied 30 eyes of 30 consecutive patients who underwent cataract surgery after LASIK for myopia. Only one type of IOL (AQ-110NV) was used for each eligible case; one eye was used per patient; and, for cases in which surgery was performed on both eyes, the eye of the previously operated eye was included. All patients did not have relevant historical data. Table 1 shows the patient parameters.

The axial length (L) and K readings were measured with the IOL master partial coherence interferometer device (Carl Zeiss Meditec, Jena, Germany) in all of the cases. Corneal topography using the Pentacam Scheimpflug system was performed before cataract surgery for each patient. The ratio between the anterior and posterior radii of the corneal curvature, which were the averages of the central radii of the steep and flat meridians in the 3.0 mm zone measured with the Pentacam Scheimpflug system, respectively, was defined as the anterior–posterior (A–P) ratio. The estimated corneal power before corneal refractive surgery (Kpre) in the double-K method was 43.86 D according to the American Society of

Cataract and Refractive Surgery (ASCRS) calculator (https://iolcalc.ascrs.org/, accessed on 20 June 2021), and the K readings of the IOL master were used as the K value after corneal refractive sur-gery (Kpost). The IOL power calculation used the double-K method based on the SRK/T formula with Kpre and Kpost, as mentioned earlier. The double-K method was calculated by entering the data into a spreadsheet software (Microsoft Excel):

$$\text{Predicted postoperative refraction} = \frac{1000 n_a \left(n_a r_{post} - (n_c - 1) LOPT \right) - LP(LOPT - ACD_{est})\left(n_a r_{post} - (n_c - 1) ACD_{est} \right)}{n_a \left(V(n_a r_{post} - (n_c - 1) LOPT) + LOPTr_{post} \right) - 0.001 LP(LOPT - ACD_{est})\left(V(n_a r_{post} - (n_c - 1) ACD_{est}) + ACD_{est} r_{post} \right)} \quad (1)$$

where n_a is the refractive index of intraocular media (1.336), r_{post} is the radius of curvature of the anterior corneal surface measured by IOL master (r_{post} = 337.5/Kpost), n_c is the refractive index of the cornea (1.333), $LOPT$ is the adjusted axial length considering that is measured with optical biometry (L + 0.65696 − 0.02029 L), LP is the implanted IOL power, and ACD_{est} is the ELP (named ACD_{est} in the original publication [6,7]) of the double-K method. ACD_{est} is calculated from corneal height in mm and Offset, where the corneal height is calculated using Kpre (43.86D); offset is calculated from A constants.

Table 1. Parameters of patients who underwent cataract surgery after corneal refractive surgery used for obtaining the regression formula to estimate the C-factor of the ISS method.

Parameter	Post-LASIK (n = 30) Mean ± SD (Range)
Age (years)	55.4 ± 10.3 (22–71)
Axial length (mm)	26.75 ± 1.67 (24.81–29.63)
Mean K by IOL master (D) Mean corneal radius of curvature by IOL master (mm) (keratometric index = 1.3375)	38.90 ± 2.35 (33.08–41.88) 8.68 ± 0.56 (8.06–10.20)
Mean anterior corneal radius of curvature by Pentacam (mm)	8.73 ± 0.58 (7.97–10.45)
Mean posterior corneal radius of curvature by Pentacam (mm)	6.33 ± 0.26 (5.71–6.88)

K = keratometric readings; D = diopter; LASIK = laser in situ keratomileusis.

The prediction errors were calculated by subtracting the predicted postoperative refraction from the postoperative manifest refraction (spherical equivalent) 1 month after cataract surgery. The prediction error and A–P ratio were plotted on a scattergram (Figure 1). The two parameters were significantly correlated (Pearson correlation coefficient, $R = 0.678$, $p < 0.001$), and the best-fit regression equation was obtained as follows:

$$y = 3.28 x - 4.00. \quad (2)$$

The predicted refraction error obtained from this regression equation was defined as the correction factor (C-factor):

$$\text{C-factor} = 3.28 \times \text{A-P ratio} - 4.00. \quad (3)$$

The ISS method corrects the target refraction value of the double-K method based on the SRK/T formula by adding the C-factor (C). The predicted refraction by the ISS method is expressed as follows:

$$\text{Predicted postoperative refraction by the ISS method} = \frac{1000 n_a \left(n_a r_{post} - (n_c - 1) LOPT \right) - LP(LOPT - ACD_{est})\left(n_a r_{post} - (n_c - 1) ACD_{est} \right)}{n_a \left(V(n_a r_{post} - (n_c - 1) LOPT) + LOPTr_{post} \right) - 0.001 LP(LOPT - ACD_{est})\left(V(n_a r_{post} - (n_c - 1) ACD_{est}) + ACD_{est} r_{post} \right)} + C \quad (4)$$

The IOL power for the desired refraction using the ISS method is obtained as follows

$$L power\ for\ the\ desired\ refraction\ using\ the\ ISS\ method \\ = \frac{1000 n_a \left(n_a r_{post} - (n_c-1) LOPT - 0.001(DR-C)\left(V\left(n_a r_{post}-(n_c-1)LOPT\right)+LOPT\ r_{post}\right)\right)}{(LOPT-ACD_{est})\left(n_a r_{post}-(n_c-1)ACD_{est}-0.001(DR-C)\left(V\left(n_a r_{post}-(n_c-1)ACD_{est}\right)+ACD_{est} r_{post}\right)\right)} \quad (5)$$

where DR is the desired refraction after cataract surgery, C is the C-factor, and V is the vertex distance (12 mm).

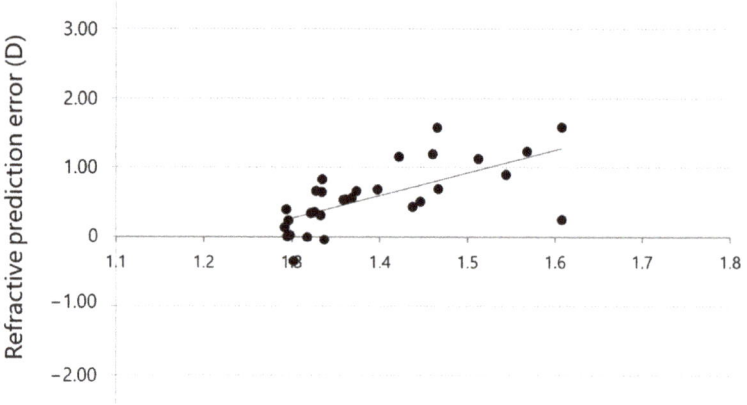

Figure 1. Correlation between the anterior–posterior ratio of corneal radii and refractive prediction error (Pearson correlation coefficient, R = 0.678, $p < 0.001$).

2.4. Intraocular Lens Power Calculations Using the ISS Method and Comparison of the Predictability of the ISS Method with That of Other Formulas or Methods

Fifty-nine eyes of 59 consecutive patients in another group who underwent cataract surgery after the group studied in item 2.3 were included in the study. Table 2 shows the patient parameters. The IOL power was calculated using the ISS method. The postoperative refraction (manifest refraction) was obtained 1 month after cataract surgery.

The predictability of the ISS method was compared with the Shammas no-history method [15,22], Haigis-L formula [24], Potvin–Hill pentacam method [25], and Barrett True K no-history formula [28,29]. These IOL calculation formulas or methods do not require preoperative data and were performed using the ASCRS IOL power calculator.

The prediction refractive error was calculated from the difference between the actual postoperative manifest refraction and the predicted refraction for each formula or method. The mean numerical error; median absolute error; mean absolute error; and percentages of eyes within ±0.25, ±0.50, and ±1.00 D of the target refraction were compared among formulas and methods.

2.5. Statistical Analyses

We conducted statistical analyses using commercially available statistical software (BellCurve for Excel, Social Survey Research Information Co., Ltd., Tokyo, Japan). The relationship between two sets of data was analyzed using Pearson correlation coefficient test. The one-sample t-test was used to assess whether the mean numerical refraction prediction errors produced by the various methods were significantly different from zero. The Wilcoxon signed-rank test was used to compare the absolute predicted refractive error with the ISS-method and with the other formulas. The percentages of eyes within ±0.25, ±0.50, and ±1.00 D of the target correction were compared with the ISS method and other calculation methods using the Fisher exact test. The Bonferroni correction was applied for multiple tests. The results were expressed as mean ± standard deviation, and values of $p < 0.05$ were considered statistically significant.

Table 2. Parameters in patients who underwent cataract surgery after LASIK in comparing the predictability of the various formulas ($n = 59$).

	Mean ± SD (Range)
Age (years)	59.0 ± 9.3 (36–77)
Axial length (mm)	27.01 ± 1.94 (23.99–32.76)
Mean K by IOL master (D) Mean corneal radius of curvature by IOL master (mm)(keratometric index = 1.3375)	38.95 ± 2.54 (33.84–43.25) 8.66 ± 0.57 (7.80–9.97)
Mean anterior corneal radius of curvature by Pentacam (mm)	8.68 ± 0.55 (7.81–9.86)
Mean posterior corneal radius of curvature by Pentacam (mm)	6.36 ± 0.29 (5.70–7.31)
TNP (4.0 mm) by Pentacam (D)	37.30 ± 2.55 (31.60–41.80)

K = keratometric readings; D = diopter; LASIK = laser in situ keratomileusis, TNP = true net power.

3. Results

The mean values of the numerical and absolute prediction errors using the ISS method were -0.02 ± 0.45 D (range, -1.11 to 0.96 D) and 0.35 ± 0.27 D (range, 0.01 to 1.11 D), respectively. The median value of the absolute prediction errors was 0.29 D. The prediction errors using the ISS method were within ±0.25 D in 29 eyes (49.2%), ±0.50 D in 45 eyes (76.3%), and ±1.00 D in 57 eyes (96.6%).

Figure 2 shows the distributions of the prediction errors. Table 3 shows the numerical and absolute prediction errors of the targeted refraction retrospectively when various formulas were used. In terms of numerical prediction errors, the Shammas no-history method showed a statistically significant difference from zero and myopic shift. In terms of median absolute error, the ISS method median absolute error was significantly lower than those of Shammas no-history method ($p = 0.028$) and Potvin–Hill pentacam methods ($p = 0.025$).

Figure 3 shows the percentages of eyes within ±0.25, ±0.50, and ±1.00 D from the target refraction. There were no statistically significant differences between the groups.

Table 3. The refractive prediction error of the targeted refraction using the various formulas.

Formula/Method	Refractive Prediction Error (D)				
	Numerical		Absolute		
	Mean ± SD (Range)	p-Value	Mean ± SD (Range)	Median	p-Value vs. ISS
ISS	−0.02 ± 0.45 (−1.11–0.96)	0.770	0.35 ± 0.27 (0.01–1.11)	0.29	N/A
Shammas	−0.20 ± 0.54 (−1.42–1.36)	0.005 *	0.45 ± 0.36 (0.00–1.42)	0.29	0.028 *
Haigis-L	0.07 ± 0.59 (−1.26–1.59)	0.361	0.45 ± 0.38 (0.00–1.59)	0.37	0.199
Potvin–Hill	0.13 ± 0.65 (−1.05–2.34)	0.124	0.50 ± 0.43 (0.02–2.34)	0.38	0.025 *
Barrett True K	0.02 ± 0.58 (−1.16–1.61)	0.754	0.43 ± 0.39 (0.03–1.61)	0.28	0.581

* $p < 0.05$. ISS = Iida–Shimizu–Shoji method, Shammas = Shammas no-history method, Haigis-L = Haigis-L formula, Potvin–Hill = Potvin–Hill pentacam method, Barrett True K = Barrett True K no-history formula.

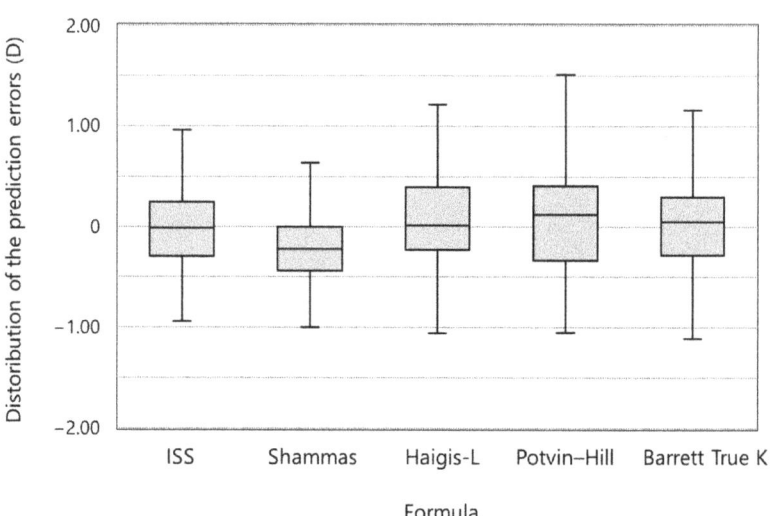

Figure 2. Intraocular lens power prediction errors using various methods (ISS = Iida–Shimizu–Shoji method; Shammas = Shammas no-history method; Haigis-L = Haigis-L formula; Potvin–Hill = Potvin–Hill pentacam method; Barrett True K = Barrett True K ho-history formula).

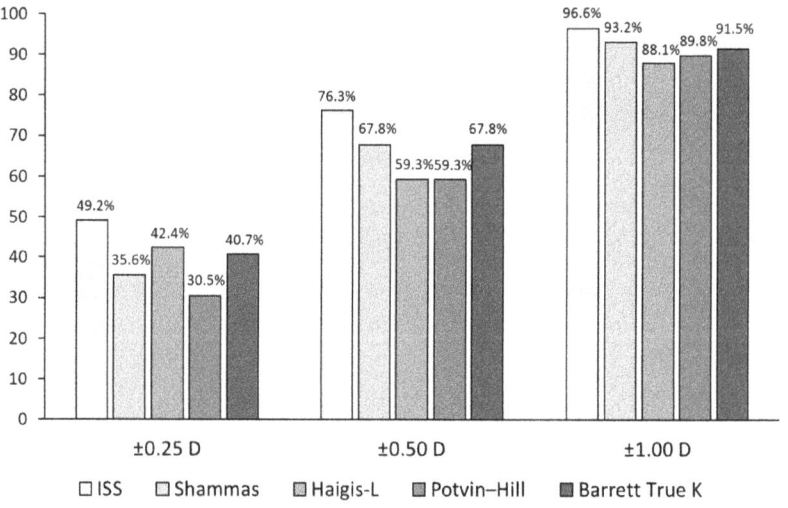

Figure 3. Comparison of the percentages of eyes within ±0.25, ±0.50, and ±1.00 D from the target refraction between IOL power calculation formulas (ISS = Iida–Shimizu–Shoji method; Shammas = Shammas no-history method; Haigis-L = Haigis-L formula; Potvin–Hill = Potvin–Hill pentacam method; Barrett True K = Barrett True K no-history formula).

4. Discussion

In this study, we examined the predictability of the ISS method, a no-history method we devised, and the formula for post-refractive surgery that can be calculated with the ASCRS calculator. The predictability of the ISS method was not only comparable to that of other formulas, but also better than that of some other formulas.

The principle of the ISS method is simple: the predicted refractive value is calculated using the C-factor, which is calculated from the correlation between the refractive error obtained by the double-K method and the A–P ratio of the radius of curvature of the cornea.

Preoperative data are required for Kpre, which is used in the double-K method, and Kpost must be obtained using the clinical history method, but if preoperative data are sometimes not available, the calculation cannot be performed. When selecting preoperative and postoperative data, care should be taken to select the timing of the data. Refractive changes not only in the cornea, but also in the lens may be included in the data. Wang et al. reported that the no-history method had better predictability than the method using preoperative data or changes in refractive values before and after refractive surgery [30].

Each of the no-history methods available in the ASCRS calculator has the following characteristics: the Shammas no-history method uses regression analysis to estimate corneal power after LASIK/PRK by adjusting the K measurement (Kpost), and the Kpost is the average K value from the IOLMaster. The Shammas-PL formula is used for IOL power calculation [15,22]. The Haigis-L formula takes the corneal radius measured by the IOLMaster and generates a corrected corneal radius using the Haigis-L algorithm, which is then used in the normal Haigis formula to calculate the IOL power after myopic laser vision correction [24]. The Potvin–Hill pentacam method uses regression analysis to estimate corneal power after LASIK/PRK using the TNP_Apex_Zone40 values from pentacam and values for ocular axial length and anterior chamber depth (if available). This method uses the Shammas-PL formula to calculate IOL power [25]. The Barrett True-K formula uses the Universal II formula, which is a modification of the original Universal Theory formula [28]. The other is the "True-K no-history formula", which is calculated only from data obtained when the patient undergoes cataract surgery. Details regarding the design of the True-K and Universal II formulas have not been released.

In the present study, the numeric refractive prediction error of the Shammas no-history method was significantly far from 0 D and myopic shifted, and the absolute refractive prediction error was significantly larger in the Shammas no-history method and Potvin–Hill pentacam methods than in the ISS method. As the Shammas-PL formula was used to calculate IOL power in the Potvin–Hill pentacam method, it is possible that these two formulas caused the significant difference.

In comparison with the figures in the literature, in 104 eyes with previous LASIK, Wang et al. reported that the median absolute refractive prediction error of 0.39 D for Haigis-L, 0.48 D for Shammas, and 0.42 D for Barrett True-K [31]. In 246 eyes with previous LASIK/PRK, Ianchulev et al. reported a median absolute refractive error of 0.53 D for Haigis-L and 0.51 D for Shammas [32]. In 58 eyes with previous LASIK/PRK, Abulafia et al. reported a median absolute refractive error of 0.46 D for Shammas, 0.58 D for Haigis-L, and 0.33 D for Barrett True-K [29]. Our study showed better results than these reports, but this difference is probably due to differences in the population groups studied and whether or not the type of IOL was standardized.

Although the formula is not included in the ASCRS calculator, as a calculation method using the same pentacam and using the anterior–posterior surface of the corneal radius of curvature, Saiki et al. focused on the fact that the posterior corneal surface data did not change before and after excimer laser corneal refractive surgery and developed the posterior corneal curvature radius; they developed the A-P method to estimate Kpre before corneal refractive surgery based on the radius [26,27]. However, even if the preoperative K value can be predicted, as long as the third-generation IOL power formula involving K value is used to calculate ELP, it is known that the use of K value to calculate ELP can be one of the causes of refractive error even in cases without refractive surgery [33], so refractive may contain at least the same amount of refractive error factors as cataract cases that have not undergone surgery.

The ISS method uses a constant value of 43.86 D as Kpre, which is used in the ASCRS calculator. Although accurate prediction of ELP is difficult, setting Kpre to a constant value in the ISS method reduces the effect on the K value on the refractive error characteristic of the third-generation IOL power calculation formula, because the K value is involved in the calculation of ELP, and this may be one of the reasons the refractive error becomes smaller.

There are limitations to this study. The main limitation is the small sample size. The C factor used in the ISS method was calculated using a regression equation, but only 30 eyes were subject to this regression equation for post-LASIK cataract surgery cases. However, we believe that we were able to eliminate the influence of internal correlation by targeting one eye per case and that of refractive error by the type of IOL by limiting to one type of IOL. In addition, by increasing the number of cases in the regression equation in the future, we may be able to adjust the C-factor and further improve the prediction accuracy. The number of cases in the group that compared the ISS method with the other methods was 59 eyes, but they were consecutive cases that were completely different from the cases used in the regression equation for determining the C-factor; in addition, like the cases in the regression equation, they were limited to one person, one eye, and one type of IOL.

In conclusion, multiple calculation methods are available for calculating the IOL power after refractive surgery, and it is necessary to select an IOL by calculating from multiple options. The no-history method can be calculated in all the cases, including those with preoperative data, and the ISS method can be useful for calculating the IOL power in eyes that have undergone cataract surgery after LASIK.

Author Contributions: Conceptualization, Y.I. and K.S.; Data curation, Y.I.; Formal analysis, Y.I.; Investigation, Y.I. and K.S.; Methodology, Y.I., K.S. and N.S.; Writing—original draft, Y.I.; Writing—review and editing, Y.I., K.S. and N.S. All authors have read and agreed to the published version of the manuscript.

Funding: This research received no external funding.

Institutional Review Board Statement: The study was conducted according to the guidelines of the Declaration of Helsinki and approved by the Institutional Review Board at the Kitasato University (protocol code B17-292) in 2018.

Informed Consent Statement: Informed consent was obtained from all subjects involved in the study.

Data Availability Statement: The data presented in this study are available on request from the corresponding author.

Conflicts of Interest: The authors declare no conflict of interest.

References

1. Hoffer, K.J. Intraocular lens power calculation for eyes after refractive keratotomy. *J. Refract. Surg.* **1995**, *11*, 490–493. [CrossRef]
2. Seitz, B.; Langenbucher, A.; Nguyen, N.X.; Kus, M.M.; Küchle, M. Underestimation of intraocular lens power for cataract surgery after myopic photorefractive keratectomy. *Ophthalmology* **1999**, *106*, 693–702. [CrossRef]
3. Gimbel, H.V.; Sun, R.; Kaye, G.B. Refractive error in cataract surgery after previous refractive surgery. *J. Cataract Refract. Surg.* **2000**, *26*, 142–144. [CrossRef]
4. Gimbel, H.V.; Sun, R.; Furlong, M.T.; van Westenbrugge, J.A.; Kassab, J. Accuracy and predictability of intraocular lens power calculation after photorefractive keratectomy. *J. Cataract Refract. Surg.* **2000**, *26*, 1147–1151. [CrossRef]
5. Gimbel, H.V.; Sun, R. Accuracy and predictability of intraocular lens power calculation after laser in situ keratomileusis. *J. Cataract Refract. Surg.* **2001**, *27*, 571–576. [CrossRef]
6. Retzlaff, J.A.; Sanders, D.R.; Kraff, M.C. Development of the SRK/T intraocular lens implant power calculation formula. *J. Cataract Refract. Surg.* **1990**, *16*, 333–340. [CrossRef]
7. Aramberri, J. Intraocular lens power calculation after corneal refractive surgery, double-K method. *J. Cataract Refract. Surg.* **2003**, *29*, 2063–2068. [CrossRef]
8. Holladay, J.T. Cataract Surgery in patients with previous keratorefractive surgery (RK, PRK and LASIK). *Ophthalmic Pract.* **1997**, *15*, 238–244.
9. Hugger, P.; Kohnen, T.; LaRosa, F.A.; Holladay, J.T.; Koch, D.D. Comparison of changes in manifest refraction and corneal power after photorefractive keratectomy. *Am. J. Ophthalmol.* **2000**, *129*, 68–75. [CrossRef]
10. Feiz, V.; Mannis, M.J.; Garcia-Ferrer, F.; Kandavel, G.; Darlington, J.K.; Kim, E.; Caspar, J.; Wang, J.-L.; Wang, W. Intraocular lens power calculation after laser in situ keratomileusis for myopia and hyperopia; a standardized approach. *Cornea* **2001**, *20*, 792–797. [CrossRef]
11. Hamed, A.M.; Wang, L.; Misra, M.; Koch, D.D. A comparative analysis of five methods of determining corneal refractive power in eyes that have undergone myopic laser in situ keratomileusis. *Ophthalmology* **2002**, *109*, 651–658. [CrossRef]

22. Keller, P.R.; McGhee, C.N.J.; Weed, K.H. Fourier analysis of corneal topography data after photorefractive keratectomy. *J. Cataract Refract. Surg.* **1998**, *24*, 1447–1455. [CrossRef]
23. Celikkol, L.; Pavlopoulos, G.; Weinstein, B.; Celikkol, G.; Feldman, S.T. Calculation of intraocular lens power after radial keratotomy with computerized videokeratography. *Am. J. Ophthalmol.* **1995**, *120*, 739–750. [CrossRef]
24. Rosa, N.; Capasso, L.; Romano, A. A new method of calculating intraocular lens power after photorefractive keratectomy. *J. Refract. Surg.* **2002**, *18*, 720–724. [CrossRef] [PubMed]
25. Shammas, H.J.; Shammas, M.C.; Garabet, A.; Kim, J.H.; Shammas, A.; LaBree, L. Correcting the corneal power measurements for intraocular lens power calculations after myopic laser in situ keratomileusis. *Am. J. Ophthalmol.* **2003**, *36*, 426–432. [CrossRef]
26. Wang, L.; Booth, M.A.; Koch, D.D. Comparison of intraocular lens power calculation methods in eyes that have undergone LASIK. *Ophthalmology* **2004**, *111*, 1825–1831. [CrossRef]
27. Camellin, M.; Calossi, A. A new formula for intraocular lens power calculation after refractive corneal surgery. *J. Refract. Surg.* **2006**, *22*, 187–199. [CrossRef]
28. Masket, S.; Masket, S.E. Simple regression formula for intraocular lens power adjustment in eyes requiring cataract surgery after excimer laser photoablation. *J. Cataract Refract. Surg.* **2006**, *32*, 430–434. [CrossRef]
29. Walter, K.A.; Gagnon, M.R.; Hoopes, P.C., Jr.; Dickinson, P.J. Accurate intraocular lens power calculation after myopic laser in situ keratomileusis, bypassing corneal power. *J. Cataract Refract. Surg.* **2006**, *32*, 425–429. [CrossRef] [PubMed]
30. Borasio, E.; Stevens, J.; Smith, G.T. Estimation of true corneal power after keratorefractive surgery in eyes requiring cataract surgery: BESSt formula. *J. Cataract Refract. Surg.* **2006**, *32*, 2004–2014. [CrossRef]
31. Rabsilber, T.M.; Reuland, A.J.; Holzer, M.P.; Auffarth, G.U. Intraocular lens power calculation using ray tracing following excimer laser surgery. *Eye* **2007**, *21*, 697–701. [CrossRef]
32. Shammas, H.J.; Shammas, M.C. No-history method of intraocular lens power calculation for cataract surgery after myopic laser in situ keratomileusis. *J. Cataract Refract. Surg.* **2007**, *33*, 31–36. [CrossRef]
33. Einighammer, J.; Oltrup, T.; Bende, T.; Jean, B. Calculating intraocular lens geometry by real ray tracing. *J. Refract. Surg.* **2007**, *23*, 393–404. [CrossRef]
34. Haigis, W. Intraocular lens calculation after refractive surgery for myopia: Haigis-L formula. *J. Cataract Refract. Surg.* **2008**, *34*, 1658–1663. [CrossRef]
35. Potvin, R.; Hill, W. New algorithm for intraocular lens power calculations after myopic laser in situ keratomileusis based on rotating Scheimpflug camera data. *J. Cataract Refract. Surg.* **2015**, *41*, 339–347. [CrossRef] [PubMed]
36. Saiki, M.; Negishi, K.; Kato, N.; Arai, H.; Toda, I.; Torii, H.; Dogru, M.; Tsubota, K. A new central-peripheral corneal curvature method for intraocular lens power calculation after excimer laser refractive surgery. *Acta Ophthalmol.* **2013**, *91*, 133–139. [CrossRef] [PubMed]
37. Saiki, M.; Negishi, K.; Kato, N.; Ogino, R.; Arai, H.; Toda, I.; Dogru, M.; Tsubota, K. Modified double-K method for intraocular lens power calculation after excimer laser corneal refractive surgery. *J. Cataract Refract. Surg.* **2013**, *39*, 556–562. [CrossRef] [PubMed]
38. Barrett, G.D. An improved universal theoretical formula for intraocular lens power prediction. *J. Cataract Refract. Surg.* **1993**, *19*, 713–720. [CrossRef]
39. Abulafia, A.; Hill, W.E.; Koch, D.D.; Wang, L.; Barrett, G.D. Accuracy of the Barrett True-K formula for intraocular lens power prediction after laser in situ keratomileusis or photorefractive keratectomy for myopia. *J. Cataract Refract. Surg.* **2016**, *42*, 363–369. [CrossRef]
40. Wang, L.; Hill, W.E.; Koch, D.D. Evaluation of intraocular lens power prediction methods using the American Society of Cataract and Refractive Surgeons Post-Keratorefractive Intraocular Lens Power Calculator. *J. Cataract Refract. Surg.* **2010**, *36*, 1466–1473. [CrossRef] [PubMed]
41. Wang, L.; Tang, M.; Huang, D.; Weikert, M.P.; Koch, D.D. Comparison of Newer Intraocular Lens Power Calculation Methods for Eyes after Corneal Refractive Surgery. *Ophthalmology* **2015**, *122*, 2443–2449. [CrossRef] [PubMed]
42. Ianchulev, T.; Hoffer, K.J.; Yoo, S.H.; Chang, D.F.; Breen, M.; Padrick, T.; Tran, D.B. Intraoperative refractive biometry for predicting intraocular lens power calculation after prior myopic refractive surgery. *Ophthalmology* **2014**, *121*, 56–60. [CrossRef] [PubMed]
43. Iijima, K.; Kamiya, K.; Iida, Y.; Shoji, N. Comparison of Predictability Using Barrett Universal II and SRK/T Formulas according to Keratometry. *J. Ophthalmol.* **2020**, *2020*, 7625725. [CrossRef] [PubMed]

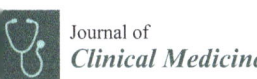

Journal of Clinical Medicine

Article

Conditional Process Analysis for Effective Lens Position According to Preoperative Axial Length

Young-Sik Yoo [1] and Woong-Joo Whang [2,*]

[1] Department of Ophthalmology, Uijeongbu St. Mary's Hospital, College of Medicine, The Catholic University of Korea, Uijeongbu-si 11765, Korea; theblue07@naver.com
[2] Department of Ophthalmology, Yeouido St. Mary's Hospital, College of Medicine, The Catholic University of Korea, Seoul 07345, Korea
* Correspondence: olokl@nate.com; Tel.: +82-2-3779-1848; Fax: +82-2-761-6869

Abstract: Purpose: To predict the effective lens position (ELP) using conditional process analysis according to preoperative axial length. Setting: Yeouido St. Mary hospital. Design: A retrospective case series. Methods: This study included 621 eyes from 621 patients who underwent conventional cataract surgery at Yeouido St. Mary Hospital. Preoperative axial length (AL), mean corneal power (K), and anterior chamber depth (ACD) were measured by partial coherence interferometry. AL was used as an independent variable for the prediction of ELP, and 621 eyes were classified into four groups according to AL. Using conditional process analysis, we developed 24 structural equation models, with ACD and K acting as mediator, moderator or not included as variables, and investigated the model that best predicted ELP. Results: When AL was 23.0 mm or shorter, the predictability for ELP was highest when ACD and K acted as moderating variables ($R2 = 0.217$). When AL was between 23.0 mm and 24.5 mm or longer than 26.0 mm, the predictability was highest when K acted as a mediating variable and ACD acted as a moderating variable ($R2 = 0.217$ and $R2 = 0.401$). On the other hand, when AL ranged from 24.5 mm to 26.0 mm, the model with ACD as a mediating variable and K as a moderating variable was the most accurate ($R2 = 0.220$). Conclusions: The optimal structural equation model for ELP prediction in each group varied according to AL. Conditional process analysis can be an alternative to conventional multiple linear regression analysis in ELP prediction.

Keywords: axial length; conditional process analysis; effective lens position; intraocular lens power calculation

1. Introduction

The accuracy of intraocular lens (IOL) power calculation is a matter of great importance in cataract surgery [1,2]. IOL power is determined by three factors: preoperative biometric data (axial length (AL), anterior chamber depth (ACD), and mean corneal power (K)), the IOL power calculation formula, and the IOL constant [3]. Cataract surgeons have aimed to create an IOL formula for the determination of the ideal refractive outcome. The prediction of postoperative ACD or effective lens position (ELP) is the most important process in IOL power calculation, and IOL power calculation error is, for the most part, due to errors in predicting ELP [4].

Although more than 10 years have passed since the concept of the Haigis formula was introduced, it still shows high predictive accuracy [5,6]. The T2 formula, using only AL and K for ELP, shows the highest predictive accuracy [5,7]. However, there is an important limitation that the two formulas above are designed based on multiple linear regression analysis [8,9]. A multiple linear regression analysis, in principle, requires the independence of explanatory variables. However, ACD and K have significant relationships with AL, which can cause errors. Statistically, the explanatory variables used in ELP prediction are considered to have a collinearity problem [10,11].

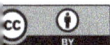

Hayes presented dozens of models in PROCESS macros for conditional process analysis [12–14]. Conditional process analysis includes not only independent variables, but also the concept of a mediating variable and a moderating variable. Using this method, we can solve the problem of multicollinearity and identify relationships between explanatory variables and develop a more accurate structural equation model for a dependent variable.

In this study, considering that the formula yielding excellent accuracy differs according to AL, we divided a total of 621 eyes into four groups according to AL. We determined the ideal model for predicting ELP in each group on the basis of conditional process analysis and the results were compared with existing IOL formula derived from a multiple linear regression analysis.

2. Materials and Methods

This retrospective case series study included 621 eyes of 621 patients who underwent uneventful and micro-coaxial phacoemulsification cataract surgery without any intraoperative complications between March 2018 and September 2019. None of the patients had a history of ocular disease, previous ocular surgery, or general disorders affecting the cornea. Exclusion criteria were amblyopia, corneal opacity, glaucoma, retinal disease, history of ocular inflammation, history of ocular trauma, and history of exposure to other intraocular surgeries. The study methods adhered to the tenets of the Declaration of Helsinki for use of human participants in biomedical research. The Institutional Review Board (IRB #SC20RASI0071) for Human Studies at Yeouido St. Mary's Hospital approved this study and informed consent was exempted by IRB of Yeouido St. Mary's Hospital.

Preoperative biometric measurements, such as K of anterior surface, ACD, and AL were obtained with an IOLMaster optical biometer (version 5, Carl Zeiss, Oberkochen, Germany) to calculate IOL power. All procedures were performed by two surgeons (H.S. Kim and W.J. Whang). All patients underwent cataract surgery through a 2.2 mm micro coaxial incision under topical anesthesia (proparacaine hydrochloride 0.5%, Alcaine, Alcon). After performing continuous curvilinear capsulorhexis with an intended diameter of 5.0 mm and hydrodissection, phacoemulsification of the nucleus was performed using an OZil torsional handpiece with the Centurion vision system (Alcon, Fort Worth, TX, USA). Following phacoemulsification, the intraocular lens (ZCB00, Johnson & Johnson Vision, Santa Ana, CA, USA) was inserted into the capsular bag using an injector and disposable cartridge system before removing the ophthalmic viscosurgical device. Finally, a balanced salt solution was injected into the corneal incision site with stromal hydration. After the surgery, postoperative antibiotic and corticosteroid eye drops were used four times daily and tapered over a month.

Subjective refraction was measured 3 months postoperatively with manifest refraction by an experienced ophthalmologist (J. Y. Lee) and ELP was back-calculated using the following thin-lens formula [15]:

$$\text{IOL power} = \frac{1336}{AL - ELP} - \frac{1336}{\frac{1336}{Z} - ELP}$$

$$Z = \frac{(nc - 1) \times 1000}{r} + \frac{1000}{\frac{1000}{PostRx} - VD}$$

where nc is the fictious corneal refractive index (1.3315), r (millimeter) is the mean value of the preoperative corneal radius, $PostRx$ is the postoperative spherical equivalent, and VD (millimeter) is the vertex distance.

The 621 eyes were stratified into 4 subgroups to investigate the appropriate structural equation model according to the preoperative AL:

1. AL $\leq$ 23.0 mm (n = 144)
2. 23.0 mm < AL $\leq$ 24.5 mm (n = 291)
3. 24.5 mm < AL $\leq$ 26.0 mm (n = 119)
4. AL > 26.0 mm (n = 67)

The ELP prediction error was defined as the value calculated by subtracting the predicted ELP from the back calculated ELP based on the thin-lens formula described above. Conditional process analysis was defined as the method for calculating ELP prediction in the present study. The accuracy of refractive outcomes (prediction error (PE), median absolute error (MedAE), and mean absolute error (MAE)) using conditional process analysis was compared to those using the Haigis formula. Refractive outcomes using the Haigis formula were calculated using an optimized IOL constant for the IOLMaster (ZCB00; $a0 = -1.302$, $a1 = 0.210$ and $a2 = 0.251$ based on ULIB site) and the zeroing of ME was performed based on the analysis methods suggested by Hoffer et al. [16]. PE was defined as the actual postoperative spherical equivalent minus the predicted spherical equivalent using the IOL power actually implanted. MedAE and MAE were the median and the average from the absolute value of the PE, respectively. The percentages of eyes with PE within ± 0.25 D, ± 0.50 D and ± 1.00 D were also obtained.

Statistical Analysis

Pearson's correlation tests were performed to determine the strength of association between AL and other variables. A multiple linear regression test was used to develop an ELP prediction equation using AL and ACD. A PROCESS macro for SPSS statistical software (version 21.0, SPSS, Inc., Chicago, IL, USA) was used for conditional process analysis. In model templates for the PROCESS macro, we chose models that consist of two or three explanatory variables. Additionally, under the assumption that the AL is the most important variable for ELP prediction, AL was set as an independent variable and ELP was set as a dependent variable. ACD and K were used as mediating variables or moderating variables, or not used. The models adopted in this study are listed in Table 1. We found the ideal combination with the highest R^2 value in 24 cases derived from 12 models in each subgroup.

Table 1. Models with 3 variables for the prediction of effective lens position (ELP). The axial length (AL) was set as an independent variable and ELP was set as a dependent variable. Each model was provided by PROCESS macro for conditional process analysis [12–14].

Model Number from PROCESS Macro [12–14]	Case	Mediating Variable	Moderating Variable
1	case 1		ACD
	case 2		K
2	case 1		ACD and K
3	case 1		ACD as a primary variable K as a secondary variable
	case 2		K as a primary variable ACD as a secondary variable
4	case 1	ACD	
	case 2	K	
	case 3	ACD and K	
5	case 1	ACD	K
	case 2	K	ACD
6	case 1	ACD as a first variable K as a second variable	
	case 2	K as a first variable ACD as a second variable	

Table 1. Cont.

Model Number from PROCESS Macro [12–14]	Case	Mediating Variable	Moderating Variable
7	case 1	ACD	K as a moderating variable for ACD
	case 2	K	ACD as a moderating variable for K
8	case 1	ACD	K as a moderating variable for ACD and ELP
	case 2	K	ACD as a moderating variable for K and ELP
14	case 1	ACD	K as a moderating variable in the process from ACD to ELP
	case 2	K	ACD as a moderating variable in the process from K to ELP
15	case 1	ACD	K as a moderating variable in the processes from ACD to ELP and from AL to ELP
	case 2	K	ACD as a moderating variable in the processes from K to ELP and from AL to ELP
58	case 1	ACD	K as a moderating variable in the processes from AL to ACD and from ACD to ELP
	case 2	K	ACD as a moderating variable in the process from AL to K and from K to ELP
59	case 1	ACD	K as a moderating variable in the processes from AL to ACD, from ACD to ELP, and from AL to ELP
	case 2	K	ACD as a moderating variable in the process from AL to K, from K to ELP, and from AL to ELP

ACD = anterior chamber depth; K = mean corneal dioptric power.

3. Results

Demographic data for a total of 621 eyes are listed in Table 2. AL ranged from 21.41 to 30.60 mm, with a mean of 24.08 ± 1.54 mm; ACD ranged from 2.02 to 4.29 mm, with a mean of 3.20 ± 0.41 mm; and K ranged from 40.30 to 49.28 diopter, with a mean of 44.12 ± 1.42 diopter. ELP ranged from 3.67 to 8.76 mm, with a mean of 5.16 ± 0.63 mm. The three preoperative parameters and ELP in the four subgroups are listed in Table 3.

Table 2. Demographic data in this study.

	Number	Mean	Min.	Max.
Axial length (mm)	621	24.08 ± 1.54	21.41	30.60
Anterior chamber depth (mm)	621	3.20 ± 0.41	2.02	4.29
Mean keratometry (diopter)	621	44.12 ± 1.42	40.30	49.28
Age	621	69.46 ± 10.20	37	98
Effective lens position (mm)	621	5.16 ± 0.63	3.67	8.76
IOL power (diopter)	621	19.98 ± 3.47	5.5	27.0
Postoperative spherical equivalent of refraction (diopter)	621	−0.85 ± 1.06	−4.13	1.00

Figure 1 shows the relationship between AL and the other two variables used in structural equation models. When all the 621 eyes were analyzed at once, AL and ACD showed a positive correlation, and AL and K showed a negative correlation (r = 0.588; $p < 0.001$ and −0.362; $p < 0.001$, respectively). However, in the subgroup analysis, both parameters showed significant correlations when AL was 24.5 mm or shorter (all $p < 0.001$).

Figure 2 demonstrates structural equation models with the highest R^2 value among 24 cases in four subgroups. When AL was shorter than 23.0 mm, the model where both

K and ACD acted as the moderating factor (Model 2 from PROCESS macro) showed the highest R^2 value (0.217, $p < 0.001$, Figure 2a). When AL ranged from 23.0 to 24.5 mm, the R^2 value (0.217, $p < 0.001$) was highest with Model 15 (K as a mediating variable, ACD as a moderating variable in both the process from AL to ELP and the process from K to ELP, Figure 2b). In the range of AL between 24.5 mm and 26.0 mm, unlike the above, when ACD acts as a mediating variable and K acts as a moderating variable in the processes of influencing ELP, the R^2 value (0.220, $p < 0.001$) is highest (Figure 2c). Figure 2d shows the model when AL was longer than 26.0 mm. The predictability is highest (R^2 value = 0.401, $p < 0.001$) with K as a mediating variable and ACD as a moderating variable.

Table 3. Demographic data in 4 subgroups classified according to preoperative axial length (AL).

		Number	Mean	Min.	Max.
AL ≤ 23.0 mm	AL (mm)	144	22.42 ± 0.39	21.41	23.00
	ACD (mm)	144	2.86 ± 0.34	2.23	3.68
	K (D)	144	45.26 ± 1.24	42.32	48.63
	ELP (mm)	144	4.75 ± 0.40	3.67	5.69
23.0 mm < AL ≤ 24.5 mm	AL (mm)	291	23.67 ± 0.41	23.01	24.50
	ACD (mm)	291	3.17 ± 0.33	2.02	4.11
	K (D)	291	43.93 ± 1.23	40.82	49.28
	ELP (mm)	291	5.02 ± 0.39	3.95	6.56
24.5 mm < AL ≤ 26.0 mm	AL (mm)	119	25.05 ± 0.37	24.51	25.99
	ACD (mm)	119	3.43 ± 0.31	2.56	4.13
	K (D)	119	43.48 ± 1.44	40.30	47.05
	ELP (mm)	119	5.38 ± 0.48	4.21	7.05
AL > 26.0 mm	AL (mm)	67	27.50 ± 1.17	26.06	30.60
	ACD (mm)	67	3.64 ± 0.30	3.01	4.29
	K (D)	67	43.64 ± 1.17	40.38	45.65
	ELP (mm)	67	6.25 ± 0.76	4.98	8.76

ACD = anterior chamber depth; K = mean corneal dioptric power; ELP = effective lens position; D = diopter.

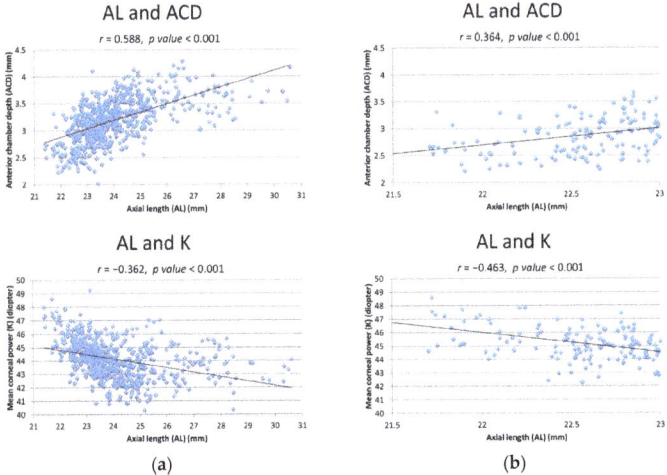

(a)   (b)

Figure 1. Cont.

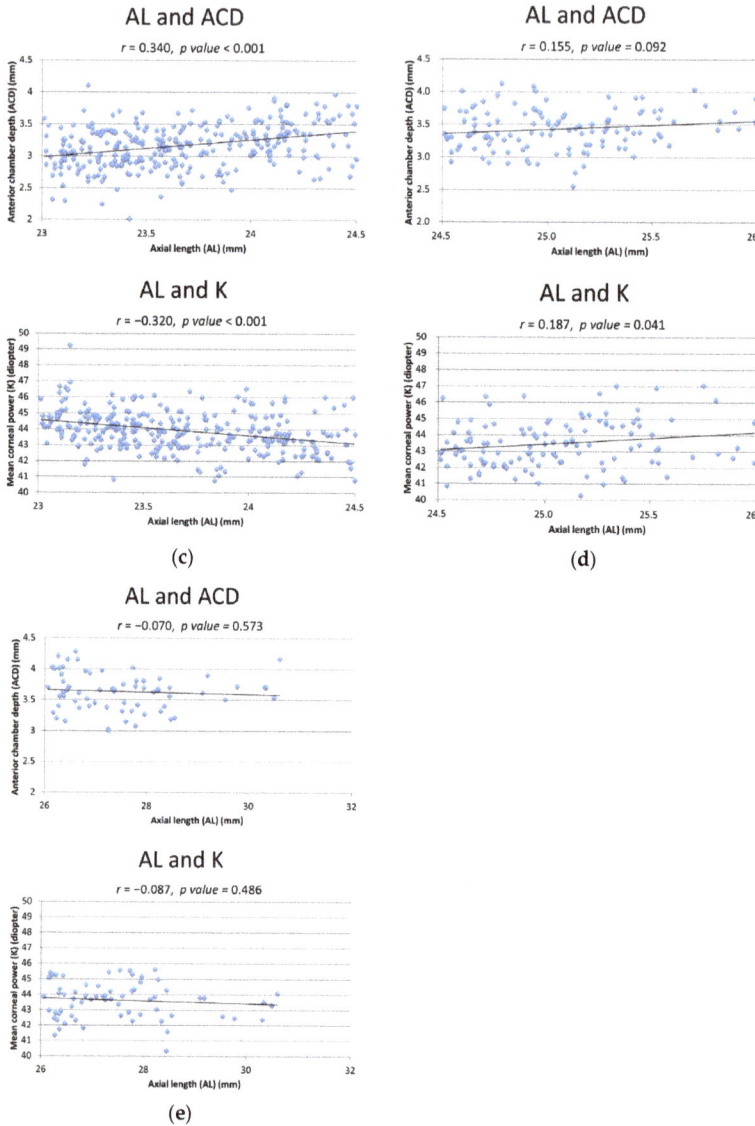

Figure 1. The relationships between axial length (AL) and other variables for structural equation models. (**a**) Total 621 eyes; (**b**) AL ≤ 23.0 mm; (**c**) 23.0 mm < AL ≤ 24.5 mm; (**d**) 24.5 mm < AL ≤ 26.0 mm; (**e**) AL > 26.0 mm. K = mean corneal dioptric power; ACD = anterior chamber depth.

Table 4 shows regression formulas derived from a multiple linear regression analysis using AL and ACD in a total of 621 eyes and conditional process analysis.

The mean ELP prediction error and the predictive accuracy from the above two analysis methods are listed in Table 5. The results from conditional process analysis yielded lower standard deviation (SD) of mean ELP prediction error, lower SD of mean prediction error, lower median absolute error and lower mean absolute error compared with results from a multiple regression test. It also produced higher percentages within ±0.25, ±0.50, and ±1.00 diopter.

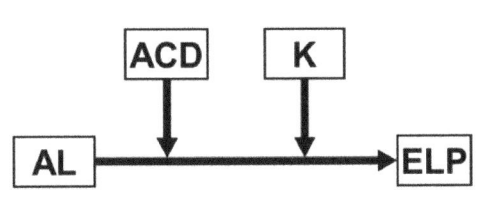

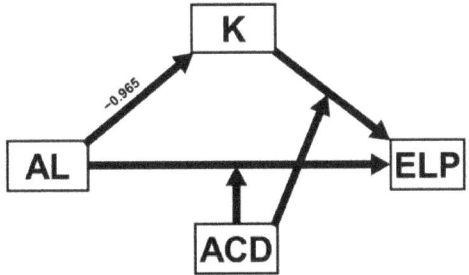

(a) (b)

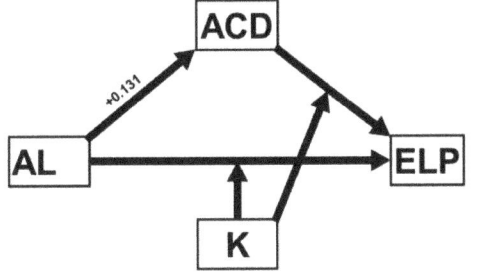

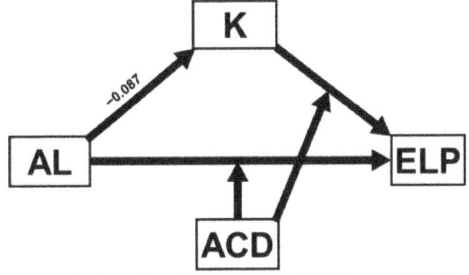

(c) (d)

Figure 2. The structural equation models for the prediction of effective lens position (ELP) in each range of axial length (AL). (a) AL ≤ 23.0 mm; (b) 23.0 mm < AL ≤ 24.5 mm; (c) 24.5 mm < AL ≤ 26.0 mm; (d) AL > 26.0 mm. K = mean corneal dioptric power; ACD = anterior chamber depth.

Table 4. Regression formulas for prediction of effective lens position according to preoperative axial length.

	Regression Formula for ELP Prediction	
	Haigis Formula	Conditional Process Analysis
AL ≤ 23.0 mm		78.662 − 3.527 × AL + 8.784 × ACD − 2.399 × K −0.393 × AL × ACD + 0.112 × AL × K
23.0 mm < AL ≤ 24.5 mm	−2.123 + 0.288 × AL + 0.107 × ACD	25.237 − 0.443 × AL − 10.495 × ACD − 0.225 × K + 0.254 × AL × ACD + 0.103 × ACD × K
24.5 mm < AL ≤ 26.0 mm		−236.636 + 10.309 × AL − 5.945 × ACD + 5.380 × K −0.231 × AL × K + 0.143 × ACD × K
AL > 26.0 mm		−49.768 + 0.870 × AL + 11.757 × ACD + 0.722 × K −0.123 × AL × ACD − 0.188 × ACD × K

ACD = anterior chamber depth; AL = axial length; K = mean corneal dioptric power; ELP = effective lens position.

Table 5. Predictive outcomes derived from the Haigis formula and conditional process analysis.

		Haigis Formula	Conditional Process Analysis
Mean ELP prediction error (D)		0.000 ± 0.424	0.000 ± 0.396
Mean prediction error (D)		0.000 ± 0.521	0.000 ± 0.488
Median absolute error (D)		0.344	0.331
Mean absolute error (D)		0.408 ± 0.324	0.386 ± 0.299
Percentages of Eyes within (D)	±0.25	39.1	39.8
	±0.50	68.6	70.9
	±1.00	94.0	95.3

ELP = effective lens position; D = diopter.

4. Discussion

The results of this study demonstrated that the optimal structural equation models, consisting of preoperative parameters for the prediction of ELP, were different according to preoperative AL. The regression equations derived from the conditional process analysis could be developed into an IOL calculation formula with high predictive accuracy.

Recently, the Barret Universal II formula, the EVO (Emmetropia Verifying Optical) formula, the Hill-RBF (radial basis function) formula, and the Kane formula have been introduced, and the accuracy of these new formulas has been reported to be improved compared to existing ones [17]. Unfortunately, the detailed mechanism of these new formulas is not known. In particular, both the Hill-RBF and the Kane formula are well known for using artificial intelligence algorithms. In addition, the possibility of IOL calculation formulas using multilayer perceptron, which is another form of artificial intelligence, has been suggested [18]. Even if the design mechanism of artificial intelligence is clearly disclosed, artificial intelligence algorithms usually have multiple hidden layers, so surgeons cannot understand the detailed calculation process [19]. This effect is called the "black box effect" and has been pointed out as a disadvantage in equations through artificial intelligence. Of course, the accuracy of IOL power calculation through artificial intelligence is already high, and there is no doubt that it will develop further in the future. However, through the results of this study, we would emphasize that the accuracy of the formula can be improved through conditional process analysis, and that the information on the detailed calculation process can be clearly provided to anyone.

The formula that produces high accuracy for postoperative refractive outcomes differs according to preoperative AL. When the AL is markedly short or long, the accuracy of the IOL calculation formula is lower than that in eyes with AL in the normal range. The Hoffer Q formula was more accurate than the other formulas in cases of eyes with short AL (AL < 22.0 mm) [20,21]. Wang et al. advocated the use of the Haigis formula for the determination of IOL power in myopia with long AL [22], so we divided a total of 621 eyes into four subgroups in 1.5 mm increments according to AL.

The correlation between postoperative refraction error and AL and K has also been studied in patients that underwent cataract surgery after refractive surgery. Recently, an advanced lens measurement approach (ALMA) was proposed to improve the accuracy of postoperative refraction error by Rosa et al. [23]. They showed the improvement of R Factor [24] and ALxK methods [25] by applying ALMA, which is a mixed theoretical regression method based on the SRK-T formula.

Almost all theoretical formulas for IOL power calculation are based on the use of a simplified eye model with a thin cornea and an IOL model. [26]. With this approach, the power of the IOL can be easily calculated using the Gauss equation in paraxial optics. [27]. ELP is back-calculated by "predicting" the effective ACD value with the actual postoperative refraction of a given data set. Therefore, ELP is formula-dependent and does not need to consider the real postoperative IOL position in terms of the eye's anatomy [28]. Models based on statistically analyzed relationships between some or all of the previously mentioned preoperative measurements of the eye and postoperative IOL position have been used to predict ELP in preoperative settings. In 1975, Fyodorov et al. [29] derived an equation based on the individual eye's keratometry and AL to estimate ELP. Third-generation formulas, including the Hoffer Q, [27] Holladay 1, [28] and SRK/T formulas, [30] use AL and K to predict ELP and IOL power calculation, and the main difference among these formulas is the predicted value of ELP. As ACD values can be measured accurately after the development of slit-scan technology, a fourth-generation formula, the Haigis formula, was developed to estimate ELP with the AL and ACD values, [31,32]. The commonality of the various formulas used from the past to the present is that the AL is considered to be the most important factor in ELP prediction. Therefore, in this study, the AL was set as a constant independent variable in the ELP prediction process.

Sheard et al. concluded that the SRK/T formula has non-physiologic behavior that contributes to IOL power prediction errors [9]. Specifically, Reitblat et al. found that the SRK/T formula induced myopic results in eyes with a mean K greater than 46.0 diopter, and hyperopic results in eyes with a mean K lower than 42.0 diopter [33]. In contrast, the Haigis formula, which does not consider corneal steepness during ELP calculation, causes myopic outcomes in flat corneas. This tendency has also been proven in large-scale research by Melles et al. [6]. However, previous studies have concluded that there is no significant association between mean K and postoperative IOL position [11,24]. In this study, we attempted to investigate the effects of K on ELP and to determine why the conclusions of the above-mentioned studies are controversial. We found a highly predictable model by setting K as variables that mediate or moderate the action of AL.

In general, ACD is positively correlated with AL, and this was reconfirmed in this study. In other words, ACD and AL inevitably have the problem of multicollinearity. However, the results of this study documented the correlation between the two parameters varies depending on the range of AL. ACD, like K, also acted as a mediator or a moderator depending on the AL and has been found to be an essential element in ELP prediction.

There are some limitations in this study. We did not evaluate other factors such as lens thickness (LT) or corneal diameter. Recently, there has been a growing interest in the thickness of the crystalline lens and LT is considered in newly developed IOL power calculation formulas. Norrby et al. concluded that LT was not an essential factor and ACD alone would predict the postoperative IOL position accurately [11]. In the above study, they used a partial least squares (PLS) regression test and LT, as an independent variable, may not be as effective. However, it could act as a factor that mediates or modulates the effect of ACD, and it is also expected that this will further improve the accuracy of the equation. Corneal diameter was significantly correlated with postoperative IOL position in another study [34]. Therefore, it is thought that corneal diameter can act as a mediator in the process from AL to ELP by itself (direct effect), or can act as a factor that mediates or moderates the effect of K (indirect effect). Corneal asphericity is another candidate. The prediction error from modern IOL calculation formulas was influenced by corneal asphericity [35,36]. Corneal asphericity could be a mediating or moderating variable in the process where K or corneal diameter affects ELP. Various models have already been introduced that can handle many variables using conditional process analysis. If new variables are included in conditional process analysis, the predictive accuracy of the equation would be further improved. A second limitation is the relatively small population. The main problem that can arise from the small population is the overfitting of the derived equation. This "overfitting" problem would be solved by increasing the number of the study populations in future studies. In addition, ideal models were found by classifying four groups in 1.5 mm increments in this study. If the number of populations is sufficient, we can find more optimized models by reducing the units of AL and increasing the number of subgroups. Lastly, the analysis of refractive outcomes based on postoperative refraction could be affected by the bias in the preoperative measurement of AL, as shown by the decrease in AL measured using an IOLMaster after cataract surgery reported by De Bernardo M et al. [37].

In conclusion, depending on the preoperative AL, the ideal structural equation model for ELP prediction derived from conditional process analysis differs. Conditional process analysis can be an alternative to conventional multiple linear regression analysis in ELP prediction and IOL power calculation.

4.1. What Was Known

- The formula that produces high accuracy for postoperative refractive outcomes differs according to preoperative axial length.
- The prediction of effective lens position is the most important process in modern IOL calculation formulas.

4.2. What This Parer Adds

- In conditional process analysis, the ideal model for the prediction of effective lens position varies according to preoperative axial length.
- Structural equation modeling from conditional process analysis is an effective tool for the prediction of an effective lens position.

Author Contributions: Conceptualization, Y.-S.Y. and W.-J.W.; methodology, Y.-S.Y. and W.-J.W.; software, W.-J.W.; validation, Y.-S.Y. and W.-J.W.; formal analysis, W.-J.W.; investigation, W.-J.W.; resources, W.-J.W.; data curation, Y.-S.Y. and W.-J.W.; writing—original draft preparation, Y.-S.Y. and W.-J.W.; writing—review and editing, Y.-S.Y. and W.-J.W.; visualization, Y.-S.Y. and W.-J.W.; supervision, W.-J.W.; project administration, W.-J.W.; funding acquisition, Y.-S.Y. All authors have read and agreed to the published version of the manuscript.

Funding: This research was supported by Basic Science Research Program through the National Research Foundation of Korea (NRF) funded by the Ministry of Education (2021R1I1A1A01056094).

Institutional Review Board Statement: The study was conducted in accordance with the Declaration of Helsinki and approved by the Institutional Review Board (IRB #SC20RASI0071) for Human Studies at Yeouido St. Mary's Hospital.

Informed Consent Statement: Patient consent was waived due to the design of the present study (retrospective study) by IRB of Yeouido St. Mary's Hospital.

Data Availability Statement: Data collected for this study, including individual patient data, will not be made available.

Conflicts of Interest: The authors declare no conflict of interest.

References

1. Kershner, R.M. Clear corneal cataract surgery and the correction of myopia, hyperopia, and astigmatism. *Ophthalmology* **1997**, *104*, 381–389. [CrossRef]
2. Kohnen, T.; Koch, M.J. Refractive aspects of cataract surgery. *Curr. Opin. Ophthalmol.* **1998**, *9*, 55–59. [CrossRef] [PubMed]
3. Drexler, W.; Findl, O.; Menapace, R.; Rainer, G.; Vass, C.; Hitzenberger, C.; Fercher, A.F. Partial coherence interferometry: A novel approach to biometry in cataract surgery. *Am. J. Ophthalmol.* **1998**, *126*, 524–534. [CrossRef]
4. Norrby, S. Sources of error in intraocular lens power calculation. *J. Cataract Refract. Surg.* **2008**, *34*, 368–376. [CrossRef]
5. Cooke, D.L.; Cooke, T.L. Comparison of 9 intraocular lens power calculation formulas. *J. Cataract Refract. Surg.* **2016**, *42*, 1157–1164. [CrossRef]
6. Melles, R.B.; Holladay, J.T.; Chang, W.J. Accuracy of Intraocular Lens Calculation Formulas. *Ophthalmology* **2018**, *125*, 169–178. [CrossRef]
7. Savini, G.; Hoffer, K.J.; Balducci, N.; Barboni, P.; Schiano-Lomoriello, D. Comparison of formula accuracy for intraocular lens power calculation based on measurements by a swept-source optical coherence tomography optical biometer. *J. Cataract Refract. Surg.* **2020**, *46*, 27–33.
8. Haigis, W. Intraocular lens calculation after refractive surgery for myopia: Haigis-L formula. *J. Cataract Refract. Surg.* **2008**, *34*, 1658–1663. [CrossRef]
9. Sheard, R.M.; Smith, G.T.; Cooke, D.L. Improving the prediction accuracy of the SRK/T formula: The T2 formula. *J. Cataract Refract. Surg.* **2010**, *36*, 1829–1834. [CrossRef]
10. Hirnschall, N.; Amir-Asgari, S.; Maedel, S.; Findl, O. Predicting the postoperative intraocular lens position using continuous intraoperative optical coherence tomography measurements. *Investig. Ophthalmol. Vis. Sci.* **2013**, *54*, 5196–5203. [CrossRef]

1. Norrby, S.; Bergman, R.; Hirnschall, N.; Nishi, Y.; Findl, O. Prediction of the true IOL position. *Br. J. Ophthalmol.* **2017**, *101*, 1440–1446. [CrossRef]
2. Hayes, A.F.; Scharkow, M. The relative trustworthiness of inferential tests of the indirect effect in statistical mediation analysis: Does method really matter? *Psychol. Sci.* **2013**, *24*, 1918–1927. [CrossRef]
3. Hayes, A.F.; Preacher, K.J. Statistical mediation analysis with a multicategorical independent variable. *Br. J. Math. Stat. Psychol.* **2014**, *67*, 451–470. [CrossRef]
4. Hayes, A.F.; Rockwood, N.J. Regression-based statistical mediation and moderation analysis in clinical research: Observations, recommendations, and implementation. *Behav. Res. Ther.* **2017**, *98*, 39–57. [CrossRef]
5. Olsen, T. Calculation of intraocular lens power: A review. *Acta Ophthalmol. Scand.* **2007**, *85*, 472–485. [CrossRef] [PubMed]
6. Hoffer, K.J.; Aramberri, J.; Haigis, W.; Olsen, T.; Savini, G.; Shammas, H.J.; Bentow, S. Protocols for studies of intraocular lens formula accuracy. *Am. J. Ophthalmol.* **2015**, *160*, 403–405. [CrossRef] [PubMed]
7. Melles, R.B.; Kane, J.X.; Olsen, T.; Chang, W.J. Update on Intraocular Lens Calculation Formulas. *Ophthalmology* **2019**, *126*, 1334–1335. [CrossRef]
8. Fernandez-Alvarez, J.C.; Hernandez-Lopez, I.; Cruz-Cobas, P.P.; Cardenas-Diaz, T.; Batista-Leyva, A.J. Using a multilayer perceptron in intraocular lens power calculation. *J. Cataract Refract. Surg.* **2019**, *45*, 1753–1761. [CrossRef]
9. Kohli, M.; Prevedello, L.M.; Filice, R.W.; Geis, J.R. Implementing Machine Learning in Radiology Practice and Research. *AJR Am. J. Roentgenol.* **2017**, *208*, 754–760. [CrossRef]
10. Gavin, E.A.; Hammond, C.J. Intraocular lens power calculation in short eyes. *Eye* **2008**, *22*, 935–938. [CrossRef] [PubMed]
11. Aristodemou, P.; Knox Cartwright, N.E.; Sparrow, J.M.; Johnston, R.L. Formula choice: Hoffer Q, Holladay 1, or SRK/T and refractive outcomes in 8108 eyes after cataract surgery with biometry by partial coherence interferometry. *J. Cataract Refract. Surg.* **2011**, *37*, 63–71. [CrossRef] [PubMed]
12. Wang, J.K.; Hu, C.Y.; Chang, S.W. Intraocular lens power calculation using the IOLMaster and various formulas in eyes with long axial length. *J. Cataract Refract. Surg.* **2008**, *34*, 262–267. [CrossRef] [PubMed]
13. Rosa, N.; Cione, F.; Pepe, A.; Musto, S.; De Bernardo, M. An Advanced Lens Measurement Approach (ALMA) in post refractive surgery IOL power calculation with unknown preoperative parameters. *PLoS ONE* **2020**, *15*, e0237990. [CrossRef]
14. Rosa, N.; Capasso, L.; Romano, A. A new method of calculating intraocular lens power after photorefractive keratectomy. *J. Refract. Surg.* **2002**, *18*, 720–724. [CrossRef] [PubMed]
15. Rosa, N.; De Bernardo, M.; Borrelli, M.; Lanza, M. New factor to improve reliability of the clinical history method for intraocular lens power calculation after refractive surgery. *J. Cataract Refract. Surg.* **2010**, *36*, 2123–2128. [CrossRef] [PubMed]
16. Shammas, H.J.; Shammas, M.C. Improving the preoperative prediction of the anterior pseudophakic distance for intraocular lens power calculation. *J. Cataract Refract. Surg.* **2015**, *41*, 2379–2386. [CrossRef]
17. Hoffer, K.J. The Hoffer Q formula: A comparison of theoretic and regression formulas. (errata, 20, 677 (1994)). *J. Cataract Refract. Surg.* **1993**, *19*, 700–712. [CrossRef]
18. Holladay, J.T.; Prager, T.C.; Chandler, T.Y.; Musgrove, K.H.; Lewis, J.W.; Ruiz, R.S. A three-part system for refining intraocular lens power calculations. *J. Cataract Refract. Surg.* **1988**, *14*, 17–24. [CrossRef]
19. Fyodorov, S.N.; Galin, M.A.; Linksz, A. Calculation of the optical power of intraocular lenses. *Investig. Ophthalmol. Vis. Sci.* **1975**, *14*, 625–628.
20. Retzlaff, J.A.; Sanders, D.R.; Kraff, M.C. Development of the SRK/T intraocular lens implant power calculation formula. (erratum, 528). *J. Cataract Refract. Surg.* **1990**, *16*, 333–340. [CrossRef]
21. Haigis, W. Occurrence of erroneous anterior chamber depth in the SRK/T formula. *J. Cataract Refract. Surg.* **1993**, *19*, 442–446. [CrossRef]
22. Haigis, W.; Lege, B.; Miller, N.; Schneider, B. Comparison of immersion ultrasound biometry and partial coherence interferometry for intraocular lens calculation according to Haigis. *Graefes Arch. Clin. Exp. Ophthalmol.* **2000**, *238*, 765–773. [CrossRef] [PubMed]
23. Reitblat, O.; Levy, A.; Kleinmann, G.; Lerman, T.T.; Assia, E.I. Intraocular lens power calculation for eyes with high and low average keratometry readings: Comparison between various formulas. *J. Cataract Refract. Surg.* **2017**, *43*, 1149–1156. [CrossRef]
24. Plat, J.; Hoa, D.; Mura, F.; Busetto, T.; Schneider, C.; Payerols, A.; Villain, M.; Daien, V. Clinical and biometric determinants of actual lens position after cataract surgery. *J. Cataract Refract. Surg.* **2017**, *43*, 195–200. [CrossRef]
25. Savini, G.; Hoffer, K.J.; Barboni, P. Influence of corneal asphericity on the refractive outcome of intraocular lens implantation in cataract surgery. *J. Cataract Refract. Surg.* **2015**, *41*, 785–789. [CrossRef] [PubMed]
26. Savini, G.; Hoffer, K.J.; Barboni, P.; Schiano Lomoriello, D.; Ducoli, P. Corneal Asphericity and IOL Power Calculation in Eyes With Aspherical IOLs. *J. Refract. Surg.* **2017**, *33*, 476–481. [CrossRef] [PubMed]
27. De Bernardo, M.; Salerno, G.; Cornetta, P.; Rosa, N. Axial Length Shortening after Cataract Surgery: New Approach to Solve the Question. *Transl. Vis. Sci. Technol.* **2018**, *7*, 34. [CrossRef] [PubMed]

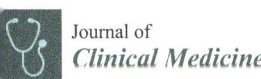

Brief Report

Facilitating Role of the 3D Viewing System in Tilted Microscope Positions for Cataract Surgery in Patients Unable to Lie Flat

Otman Sandali [1,2,*], Rachid Tahiri Joutei Hassani [3], Ashraf Armia Balamoun [4,5,6], Mohamed El Sanharawi [7] and Vincent Borderie [1]

1. Centre Hospitalier National d'Ophtalmologie des XV-XX, Pierre & Marie Curie University Paris 06, ResearchTeam 968, Institut de laVision, 75571 Paris, France; borderie@quinze-vingts.fr
2. Service de Chirurgie Ambulatoire, Hôpital Guillaume-de-Varye, 18230 Bourges, France
3. Service de Chirurgie Ambulatoire, Centre Hospitalier de Granville, 50400 Granville, France; tjhr78@hotmail.com
4. Watany Eye Hospital WEH, Cairo 11775, Egypt; ashrafarmia@gmail.com
5. Watany Research and Development Centre, Cairo 11775, Egypt
6. Ashraf Armia Eye Clinic, Giza 12655, Egypt
7. Service D'ophtalmologie, Centre Hospitalier de Châteaudun, 28200 Chateaudun, France; mohamed.elsanharawi@gmail.com
* Correspondence: sanotman1@yahoo.fr; Tel.: +33-1-40021508

Abstract: Purpose: To assess the utility of the 3D viewing system in tilted microscope positions for the performance of cataract surgery in challenging positions, for patients with difficulty remaining supine. Methods: Prospective, single-center, single-surgeon, consecutive case series of patients undergoing surgery in an inclined position. Results: 21 eyes of 15 patients who had undergone surgery at inclined positions at angles of 20° to 80°, with a mean angle of 47.62°. Surgeon comfort was considered to be globally good. The surgeon rated red reflex perception and the impression of depth as good and stable in all cases. The operating time was slightly longer for patients inclined at angles of more than 50°. On the first day after surgery, BSCVA was 20/25 or better in all cases. No ocular complications occurred in any of the interventions. Conclusions: Due to the ocular-free design of the 3D system, the surgical procedure and the positioning of the surgeon remained almost identical to that for patients undergoing surgery in a supine position, maintaining the safety of the standard surgical approach.

Keywords: cataract surgery; tilted microscope positions; 3D viewing system; patients unable to lie flat

1. Introduction

Ocular surgery is usually performed in patients lying in a supine position with the surgical microscope perpendicular to the surgical plane.

However, this usual position may not be possible if the patient cannot remain in a supine position due to medical conditions. Rotating the optical axis of the microscope perpendicular to the eye is one possible solution for such procedures in patients undergoing surgery in an inclined position [1–4]. However, it is very challenging to perform surgeries when the microscope rotation exceeds 30° in practice, because a greater rotation is incompatible with the posture of the surgeon, who needs to be able to look through the microscope oculars during surgery.

The three-dimensional (3D) digital visualization system was recently evaluated and shown to be safe for ocular surgery [5–7]. The ocular-free design of the 3D system makes it possible for the surgeon to adopt a much more ergonomic posture during surgery and may release the limitations on the axis of the microscope rotation.

In this study, we report the utility of the 3D viewing system in tilted microscope positions for cataract surgery in challenging positions in 15 consecutive patients unable to remain in a supine position.

2. Surgical Technique

This report included consecutive patients undergoing cataract surgery in an inclined position for medical reasons, at Guillaume de Varye Hospital (Bourges, France) between January 2021 and November 2021. These patients were either unable to remain in a supine position or found this position very uncomfortable. The study was approved by the ethics committee of our institution and was performed in accordance with the Declaration of Helsinki.

All the interventions were performed by the same experienced surgeon (O.S.) with the Constellation® (Alcon Surgical, Ft. Worth, TX, USA) surgical system and the 3D digital visualization system (NGENUITY®, Alcon, Fort Worth, TX, USA), connected to a (Lumera 700 Carl Zeiss Meditec, Jena, Germany) microscope.

All the operations were performed under topical anesthesia. The patients were lying in a standard reclining cataract surgical chair, the back of which was reclined to a position in which the patient felt comfortable, to ensure that the surgical conditions were good.

The surgical chair was lowered as much as possible, to ensure that the patient's eye was located at about the generator cassette level. Depending on the angle at which the patient was tilted, the microscope was tilted such that it was parallel to the eye and its optical axis was perpendicular to the surgical plane, providing good visualization (Figure 1).

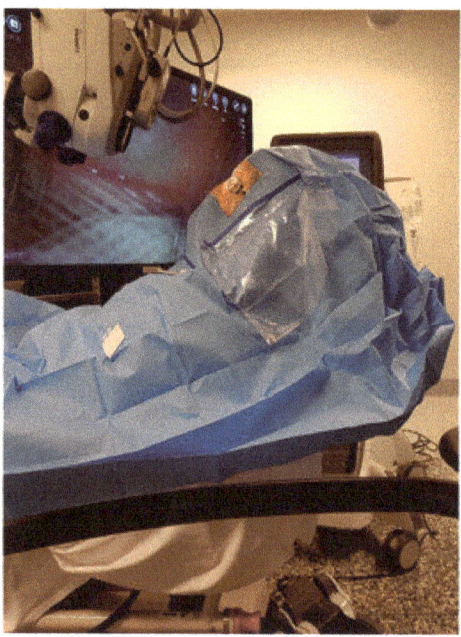

Figure 1. Patient suffering from orthopnea undergoing cataract surgery in an inclined position. The microscope was tilted perpendicular to the surgical plane.

The surgeon sat, as usual, behind the patients and a 2.2 mm principal corneal incision was made in the superotemporal quadrant for right eyes, and in the superonasal quadrant for left eyes, avoiding the eyebrow (Figure 2). The nucleus was emulsified by the divide and conquer technique (Video S1 Supplementary Material).

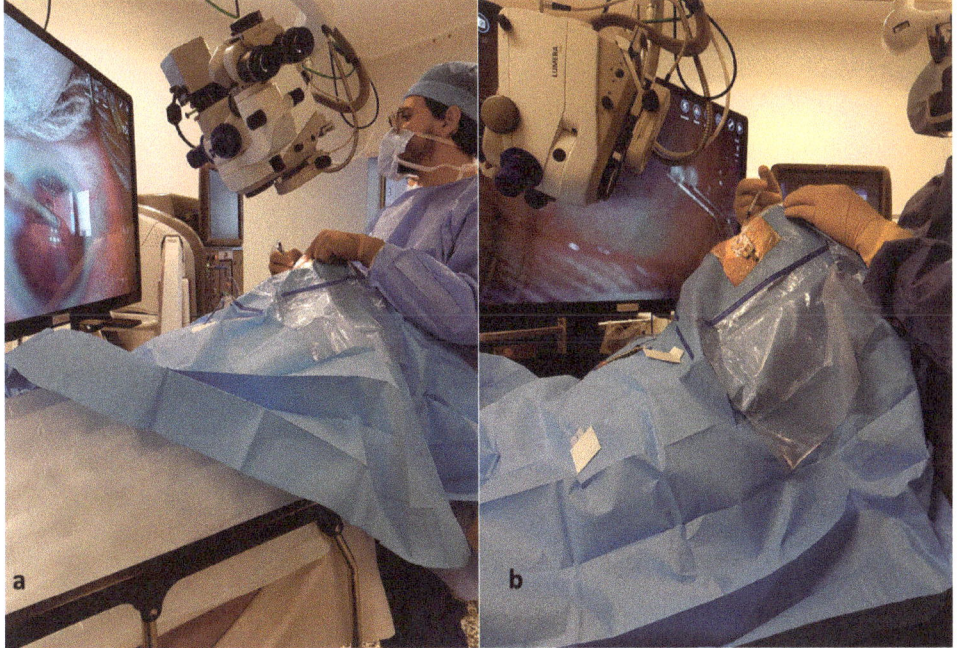

Figure 2. Surgeon positioning behind patients who underwent cataract surgery in inclined positions ((**a**): patient inclined in a 30° position. (**b**): patient inclined in a 65° position).

Pre-operative cataract grading was assessed according to a simplified nuclear classification score based on the posterior nuclear color appearance [8].

Red reflex perception, the impression of depth, the operating time, the need for corneal suture, operative complications, and surgeon comfort (scale: 1–3; 1: comfortable, 2: mild discomfort, 3: uncomfortable) were assessed with a questionnaire.

3. Results

In total, 21 eyes from 15 patients were enrolled in the study (Table 1). Most of these patients (9/15) had degenerative spinal disorders.

Table 1. Clinical characteristics and outcomes of patients who underwent cataract surgery in inclined positions.

Patient	Side	Age (Years)	Comorbidity	Cataract Grading	Preoperative BCVA	Patient Inclination (Degrees)	Surgery Duration (Minutes)	Impression of Depth	Red Reflex Perception	Surgeon Comfort *	1 Day after Surgery BCVA
1	R	91	Orthopnea	3	20/70	50	16	Good	Good	1	20/20
2	R	82	Positional Vertigo	2	20/50	40	12	Good	Good	1	20/20
2	L	82	Positional Vertigo	2	20/50	40	11	Good	Good	1	20/20
3	L	75	Back pain	4	20/100	30	10	Good	Good	1	20/25
4	R	54	Neck pain	2	20/40	45	10	Good	Good	1	20/15
4	L	54	Neck pain	2	20/50	45	12	Good	Good	1	20/15
5	R	69	Orthopnea	3	20/70	70	15	Good	Good	2	20/25
5	L	69	Orthopnea	2	20/50	70	16	Good	Good	2	20/25
6	R	72	Orthopnea	2	20/40	80	17	Good	Good	2	20/20

Table 1. Cont.

Patient	Side	Age (Years)	Comorbidity	Cataract Grading	Preoperative BCVA	Patient Inclination (Degrees)	Surgery Duration (Minutes)	Impression of Depth	Red Reflex Perception	Surgeon Comfort *	1 Day after Surgery BCVA
7	R	78	Back pain	2	20/50	60	17	Good	Good	2	20/25
8	R	80	Neck pain	2	20/50	20	9	Good	Good	1	20/25
8	L	80	Neck pain	2	20/40	20	9	Good	Good	1	20/20
9	R	59	Back pain	4	20/100	35	11	Good	Good	1	20/25
10	R	74	Orthopnea	4	20/100	65	18	Good	Good	2	20/25
11	R	83	Neck pain	3	20/70	35	10	Good	Good	1	20/25
11	L	83	Neck pain	3	20/70	35	9	Good	Good	1	20/25
12	R	75	Neck pain	2	20/50	40	12	Good	Good	1	20/15
12	L	75	Neck pain	2	20/50	40	12	Good	Good	1	20/15
13	R	81	Orthopnea	2	20/30	65	15	Good	Good	2	20/15
14	L	68	Back pain	2	20/50	55	15	Good	Good	1	20/20
15	L	77	Positional Vertigo	3	20/70	60	16	Good	Good	2	20/25

BCVA: Snellen best corrected visual acuity. * Surgeon comfort was assessed with a questionnaire (scale: 1–3, 1: comfortable, 2: mild discomfort, 3: uncomfortable).

Patients were inclined at angles of 20° to 80°, with a mean angle of 47.62°. The surgeon considered red reflex perception and the impression of depth to be good and stable in all cases, as in surgeries performed with patients lying flat. No ocular complications occurred in any of the interventions. None of the patients required corneal suture. Operating time was slightly longer for the patients inclined at angles of more than 50° ($p < 0.01$).

Surgeon comfort was rated "1" (comfortable) in all cases in which the patient was inclined at less than 60° and "2" (mild discomfort) for patients inclined at angles exceeding 60°

On the first day after surgery, BSCVA was 20/25 or better in all cases.

4. Discussion

In this series, we evaluated the facilitating role of the ocular-free design of the 3D visualization system to the performance of surgeries in unusual challenging positions using the microscope rotation, in cataract surgery on patients unable to remain supine.

Microscope tilting is used in other indications in patients undergoing operations in a supine position. Indeed, by displacing the angle of view, this technique allows the visualization of the trabecular meshwork in stent implantation or the extension of the peripheral retinal view in retinal surgery [9,10].

At high angles of standard microscope rotation, the surgeon becomes very uncomfortable and must change his posture and modify the surgical approach, sometimes even modifying the location of the incision, which may increase the risk of operative complications. In a series of 32 eyes, Richard et al. reported the results for a face-to-face upright seated position for cataract surgery in patients who cannot lie supine, with the surgeon either seated or standing, and facing the patient [2]. Inferior, temporal or inferotemporal corneal incisions were made. Capsular rupture occurred in two cases, with nucleus drop. The authors considered this surgical positioning technically challenging and recommended its use only by experienced surgeons. Muraine et al. recently reported a series of four eyes in which face-to-face phacoemulsification was performed, with a slit lamp and the surgeon sitting facing the patient and performing a temporal incision [11].

In our series of 21 eyes, due to the ocular-free design of the 3D system, the surgical procedure and the positioning of the surgeon for patients undergoing cataract surgery in an inclined position remained almost identical to that for patients undergoing surgery in a supine position. The safety of the standard surgical approach was, therefore, maintained.

Within the eye, the quality of visualization, the impression of depth and red reflex perception were considered to be very good and similar to those in standard operating conditions.

A fast and good visual recovery was recorded in all cases on the first day after surgery. The good visualization conditions and the perceived depth of field may have ensured the safety of intraocular maneuvers, accounting for this result.

In conclusion, we reported here the facilitating role of the ocular-free design of the 3D system for the performance of ocular surgery in unusual challenging positions in patients who are unable to lie flat. This system makes it possible to maintain the usual position and the safety of the standard surgical approach in such challenging conditions.

Supplementary Materials: The following supporting information can be downloaded at: https://www.mdpi.com/article/10.3390/jcm11071865/s1, Video S1: Video highlighting the surgeon's installation and the surgical procedure in a patient who underwent cataract surgery in an inclined position.

Author Contributions: O.S.: conceptualization, methodology, validation, investigation, data curation, writing–original draft preparation. R.T.J.H.: conceptualization, methodology, validation. A.A.B.: data curation, validation. M.E.S.: formal analysis, data curation. V.B.: validation, original draft preparation. All authors have read and agreed to the published version of the manuscript.

Funding: This research received no external funding.

Informed Consent Statement: Informed consent was obtained from all subjects involved in the study.

Data Availability Statement: The data that support the findings of this study are available from the corresponding author, O.S., upon request.

Conflicts of Interest: The authors declare no conflict of interest.

References

1. Ang, G.S.; Ong, J.M.; Eke, T. Face-to-face seated positioning for phacoemulsification in patients unable to lie flat for cataract surgery. *Am. J. Ophthalmol.* **2006**, *141*, 1151–1152. [CrossRef] [PubMed]
2. Lee, R.M.H.; Jehle, T.; Eke, T. Face-to-face upright seated positioning for cataract surgery in patients who cannot lie flat. *J. Cataract Refract. Surg.* **2011**, *37*, 805–809. [CrossRef] [PubMed]
3. Sohail, T.; Pajaujis, M.; Crawford, S.E.; Chan, J.W.; Eke, T. Face-to-face upright seated positioning for cataract surgery in patients unable to lie flat: Case series of 240 consecutive phacoemulsifications. *J. Cataract Refract. Surg.* **2018**, *44*, 1116–1122. [CrossRef] [PubMed]
4. Pajaujis, M.; Injarie, A.; Eke, T. Extreme face-to-face positioning for cataract surgery with patient seated upright in motorized wheelchair. *J. Cataract Refract. Surg.* **2013**, *39*, 804–805. [CrossRef] [PubMed]
5. Weinstock, R.J.; Diakonis, V.F.; Schwartz, A.J.; Weinstock, A.J. Heads-Up Cataract Surgery: Complication Rates, Surgical Duration, and Comparison with Traditional Microscopes. *J. Refract. Surg.* **2019**, *35*, 318–322. [CrossRef] [PubMed]
6. Freeman, W.R.; Chen, K.C.; Ho, J.; Chao, D.L.; Ferreyra, H.A.; Tripathi, A.B.; Nudleman, E.; Bartsch, D.U. Resolution, Depth of Field, and Physician Satisfaction during Digitally Assisted Vitreoretinal Surgery. *Retina* **2019**, *39*, 1768–1771. [CrossRef] [PubMed]
7. Sandali, O.; El Sanharawi, M.; Tahiri, J.H.R.; Roux, H.; Bouheraoua, N.; Borderie, V. Early corneal pachymetry maps after cataract surgery and influence of 3D digital visualization system in minimizing corneal oedema. *Acta Ophthal.* **2021**, *online ahead of print*. [CrossRef]
8. Mandelblum J, Fischer N, Achiron A, Goldberg M, Tuuminen R, Zunz E, Spierer O: A Simple Pre-Operative Nuclear Classification Score (SPONCS) for Grading Cataract Hardness in Clinical Studies. *J. Clin. Med.* **2020**, *29*, 3503.
9. Ohno, H. Utility of Three-Dimensional Heads-Up Surgery in Cataract And Minimally Invasive Glaucoma Surgeries. *Clin. Ophthalmol.* **2019**, *13*, 2071–2073. [CrossRef] [PubMed]
10. Sandali, O.; Tahiri, J.H.R.; Duliere, C.; El Sanharawi, M.; Borderie, V. Use of a 3D viewing system and microscope tilting to extend the peripheral retinal view. *RETINA* **2022**. [CrossRef]
11. Muraine, M.; Boutillier, G.; Toubeau, D.; Gueudry, J. Face-to-face phacoemulsification using a slitlamp in patients who are unable to lie flat. *J. Cataract Refract. Surg.* **2019**, *45*, 1535–1538. [CrossRef]

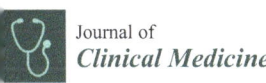

Article

Saving of Time Using a Software-Based versus a Manual Workflow for Toric Intraocular Lens Calculation and Implantation

Barbara S. Brunner [1], Nikolaus Luft [1], Siegfried G. Priglinger [1], Mehdi Shajari [1,2], Wolfgang J. Mayer [1,*] and Stefan Kassumeh [1]

[1] Department of Ophthalmology, University Hospital, LMU Munich, Mathildenstrasse 8, 80336 Munich, Germany; barbara.brunner@med.uni-muenchen.de (B.S.B.); nikolaus.luft@med.uni-muenchen.de (N.L.); siegfried.priglinger@med.uni-muenchen.de (S.G.P.); mehdi.shajari@med.uni-muenchen.de (M.S.); stefan.kassumeh@med.uni-muenchen.de (S.K.)
[2] Department of Ophthalmology, University Hospital, Theodor-Stern-Kai 7, 65933 Frankfurt, Germany
* Correspondence: wolfgang.j.mayer@med.uni-muenchen.de

Abstract: Background: To determine whether there is a significant saving of time when using a digital cataract workflow for digital data transfer compared to a manual approach of biometry assessment, data export, intraocular lens calculation, and surgery time. Methods: In total, 48 eyes of 24 patients were divided into two groups: 24 eyes were evaluated using a manual approach, whereas another 24 eyes underwent a full digital lens surgery workflow. The primary variables for comparison between both groups were the overall time as well as several time steps starting at optical biometry acquisition until the end of the surgical lens implantation. Other outcomes, such as toric intraocular lens misalignment, reduction of cylinder, surgically induced astigmatism, prediction error, and distance visual acuity were measured. Results: Overall, the total diagnostic and surgical time was reduced from 1364.1 ± 202.6 s in the manual group to 1125.8 ± 183.2 s in the digital group ($p < 0.001$). The complete time of surgery declined from 756.5 ± 82.3 s to 667.3 ± 56.3 ($p < 0.0005$). Compared to the manual approach of biometric data export and intraocular lens calculation (76.7 ± 12.3 s) as well as the manual export of the reference image to a portable external storage device (26.8 ± 5.5 s), a highly significant saving of time was achieved ($p < 0.0001$). Conclusions: Using a software-based digital approach to toric intraocular lens implantation is convenient, more efficient, and thus more economical than a manual workflow in surgery practice.

Keywords: toric intraocular lens; cataract surgery; cataract surgery workflow; efficiency; refractive surgery; refractive lens exchange; clear lens exchange

1. Introduction

The use of toric intraocular lenses (IOL) to correct corneal astigmatism has drastically changed cataract surgery over the last decade and broadened the range of indications for refractive lens exchanges [1]. The prevalence of astigmatism increases with age, with approximately 40–50% of individuals over the age of 60 years presenting a corneal astigmatism of at least 1.00 diopters (D) and thus becoming eligible for astigmatic correction using toric intraocular lenses [2,3]. In these cases, toric intraocular lenses are particularly suited to achieve postoperative independence from glasses as well as increased patient satisfaction. Not surprisingly, the implantation of toric intraocular lenses has gained massive importance in the past few years.

To enable neutralization of corneal astigmatism, a precise preoperative calculation of the toric intraocular lens power is of utmost importance [4]. The best indicator of toric intraocular lens calculation accuracy is the prediction error (PE) of residual astigmatism. Depending on the formula used to calculate toric intraocular lenses, different anatomical parameters are considered [5]. The most important parameters of all formulas are the keratometry values of the cornea since they have the greatest influence on the required toricity of IOL for neutralizing corneal astigmatism [4]. Whereas early formulas solely considered the keratometry values (K) of the anterior corneal surface, state-of-the-art formulas consider the total keratometry (TK) including the values of the anterior and posterior corneal surface. This is due to several studies stating that the posterior corneal surface significantly contributes to the total corneal astigmatism [6], and its consideration thus leads to a superior postoperative prediction accuracy [7].

A vast variety of devices mostly utilize two technologies to acquire corneal keratometry values and biometric ocular data: the rotating Scheimpflug camera and swept-source optical coherence tomography (SS-OCT). One of the most commonly used SS-OCT-based biometric devices is the IOLMaster (Carl Zeiss Meditec AG, Jena, Germany). While a predecessor version of the machine, the IOLMaster 500, was only able to measure the anterior surface of the cornea, the novel IOLMaster 700 also measures the posterior corneal curvature. With the information of the anterior and posterior corneal curvature, the IOLMaster 700 can further calculate the total refractive power of the cornea (total keratometry; TK) [8,9]. An additional feature of the IOLMaster 700 is the ability to calculate intraocular lens power onboard based on the TK values prior to surgery.

With rising numbers of toric intraocular lens implantations, especially in refractive lens exchanges, and the associated extra time effort, surgeons crave an efficient workflow and an IOL power calculation tool to keep preoperative preparation times as short as possible and intraocular lens calculation and implantation as precise as possible. Therefore, the novel cataract workflow EQ Workplace integrated in the FORUM platform (all by Carl Zeiss Meditec AG), featuring the Z CALC intraocular lens formula and calculator, was established to allow a complete digital approach from biometry assessment over the data export to intraoperative toric intraocular lens axis alignment.

To this end, this study determines whether there is a significant saving of time when using the digital cataract workflow EQ Workplace 1.6.0 within the FORUM system for digital data transfer compared to a manual approach of biometry assessment, data export, intraocular lens calculation, and surgery time using the CALLISTO eye and Z ALIGN digital tracking system.

2. Materials and Methods

This study is a prospective interventional case series performed at one single tertiary referral center in Munich, Germany (Department of Ophthalmology, University Hospital, LMU Munich, Munich, Germany). Prior to data collection and analysis, approval was obtained by the local institutional review board of the Ludwig Maximilian University (approval number: 19-731). This study complies with the criteria defined in the Declaration of Helsinki. Informed consent was given by all patients included.

The primary goal was to evaluate the saving of time when using the cataract workflow EQ Workplace 1.6.0 within the FORUM system for digital data transfer compared to a manual approach of biometry assessment, intraocular lens calculation, and effective diagnostic and surgery time using the CALLISTO eye and Z ALIGN digital tracking system. Furthermore, this case series will address the accuracy of the Z CALC 2.1.0 intraocular lens calculator (for all: Carl Zeiss Meditec AG, Jena, Germany), embedded in the EQ Workplace, in predicting intraocular lens power and postoperative spherical equivalent. In addition, diverse quality criteria were determined: the reduction of cylinder, the surgically induced astigmatism (SIA), IOL axis misalignment, and the visual outcome.

2.1. Patient Characteristics

All patients included either presented with an age-related cataract or a clear crystalline lens and a regular corneal astigmatism of at least one diopter in swept-source optical coherence tomography-based optical biometry using the IOLMaster 700 (Carl Zeiss Meditec AG). The regular corneal astigmatism was confirmed using the central corneal topography acquired with SS-OCT onboard the IOLMaster 700. Exclusion criteria were pseudo-exfoliation syndrome, irregular astigmatism, uveitis, previous vitreoretinal or refractive surgeries, other corneal pathologies, maculopathies, or ocular surface diseases. Both eyes of each study subject underwent clear lens exchange or cataract surgery. One eye received a complete digital approach starting at biometry assessment, whereas the other one underwent a manual approach. For all, phacoemulsification and toric intraocular lens implantation were performed by one experienced surgeon (W.J.M.) using a 2.4 mm clear corneal incision at 90°. To achieve intraoperative toric intraocular lens alignment, the CALLISTO eye and Z ALIGN digital tracking system utilizing a reference image assessed with the IOLMaster 700 prior to surgery, were used. All procedures and study examinations were performed at the Department of Ophthalmology, University Hospital, LMU Munich.

Three months postoperatively, manifest refraction was obtained by subjective refraction according to DIN 58220. Uncorrected and corrected distance visual acuity (UDVA and CDVA) was assessed at six meters (20 ft). Toric IOL axis alignment was evaluated with a slit lamp. To address postoperative SIA, another optical biometry was conducted.

2.2. Intraocular Lens Calculation

In all eyes, a monofocal toric (Carl Zeiss AT TORBI 709M, Carl Zeiss Meditec AG) or trifocal toric (Carl Zeiss AT LISA tri toric 939M, Carl Zeiss Meditec AG) intraocular lens with plate haptic design was implanted. The intraocular lens calculations were based on the total keratometry (TK) corneal measurements obtained by optical biometry and performed using the Z CALC intraocular lens calculator in the digital group. In the manual group, IOL were calculated onboard the IOLMaster 700 with the Haigis formula based on the TK values. Surgically induced astigmatism was implemented into the IOL calculation using the surgeon's reference SIA, calculated with the Warren Hill calculator according to previous standard lens surgeries.

2.3. Workflow Steps and Time Measurement Points

The workflow begins with optical biometry and terminates with the end of the surgical intraocular lens implantation. The effective time for all workflow steps were measured whenever the operator or/and the patient were ready for examination/surgery. Table 1 illustrates the time points/intervals of interest (Table 1).

Table 1. Workflow steps and points of interest in the manual and digital group.

Manual Group (n = 24)	Digital Group (n = 24)
Data check	EQ Workplace data check
IOL calculation (IOLMaster 700)	IOL calculation (EQ Workplace)
Export of reference image to USB memory stick	Digital reference image export via FORUM to CALLISTO eye
Import reference image to CALLISTO eye and image matching	Digital reference image import via FORUM to CALLISTO eye and image matching
IOL alignment using CALLISTO eye and Z ALIGN tracking system	
Overall surgery time	
Overall diagnostic + surgery time	

Following optical biometry, patient data was double-checked either onboard the IOLMaster 700 or in the EQ Workplace. Following the IOL calculation explained above, the reference image was either exported via a portable memory drive (USB stick) or directly transferred digitally via the EQ Workplace. After matching the reference image in the manual group, the target IOL axis had to be entered manually. The time of the reference image import as well as the image matching and IOL axis alignment are included in the overall surgery time.

2.4. Statistics and Data Analysis

Statistical analysis was performed with the open-source statistics software R (Version 4.1.2; Ross Ihaka and Robert Gentleman, R Core Team, University of Auckland, Auckland, New Zealand). Normality of data was confirmed with the Shapiro–Wilk normality test. To compare the means of time between the manual and digital group, a paired Student's t-test was performed. We considered $p < 0.01$ statistically significant. Results were reported according to the standards for reporting refractive outcomes of intraocular lens-based refractive surgery [10].

3. Results

In total, 48 eyes of 24 patients were included in the time measurement study. The mean age was 60 ± 9.8 years (range 42 to 79 years). The proportion of female eyes was 63% ($n = 30$) with 15 patients being female and nine being male. Of those eyes that received a fully digital approach, 18 eyes had a with-the-rule (WTR, axis: 60–120°) astigmatism, five eyes an against-the-rule (ATR, axis: 0–30° or 150–180°) astigmatism and one eye an oblique (axis: 30–60° or 120–150°) astigmatism.

3.1. The Digital Approach Using EQ Workplace Saves Diagnostic and Surgical Time

When the surgery was planned, patient identification, data verification in EQ Workplace as well as intraocular lens calculation and reference image export accounted for 48.0 ± 16.1 s (Table 2). Compared to the manual approach of biometric data check and intraocular lens calculation (76.7 ± 12.3 s) as well as the manual export of the reference image to a portable external storage device (26.8 ± 5.5 s), a highly significant saving of time was achieved ($p < 0.0001$).

Table 2. Time measurements at the time points of interest in the manual and digital group.

Time Point of Interest	Time, Manual Group ($n = 24$; in Seconds)	Time, Digital Group (EQ Workplace) Group ($n = 24$; in Seconds)	Level of Significance
Data check and IOL calculation	76.7 ± 12.3	48.0 ± 16.1	$p < 0.0001$
Reference image export	26.8 ± 5.5		
Reference image import and image matching	129.8 ± 18.0	54.9 ± 9.2	$p < 0.0001$
IOL alignment intraoperatively	30.7 ± 4.1	22.8 ± 5.1	$p < 0.0001$
Surgery time (overall)	756.5 ± 82.3	667.3 ± 56.3	$p < 0.0005$
Diagnostic and surgical time (overall)	1364.1 ± 202.6	1125.8 ± 183.2	$p < 0.0005$

Prior to surgery, the import of the reference image to the CALLISTO eye-tracking system and matching the same with the patient's eye took 129.8 ± 18.0 s in the manual and 54.9 ± 9.2 s in the digital group ($p < 0.0001$).

During surgery, intraocular lens alignment was significantly faster using the fully digital approach with 22.8 ± 5.1 s, compared to the manual group (30.7 ± 4.1 s; $p < 0.0001$).

Overall, the complete time of surgery was reduced from 756.5 ± 82.3 s to 667.3 ± 56.3 s using a full EQ Workplace and CALLISTO eye-tracking system approach ($p < 0.0005$; Table 2). The total diagnostic and surgical time came in as 1364.1 ± 202.6 s in the manual group and as 1125.8 ± 183.2 s in the digital group respectively ($p < 0.001$; Table 2).

3.2. Reduction of Cylinder Postoperatively

Following implantation of a toric intraocular lens in the digital group calculated with Z CALC, the mean cylinder of all 24 eyes was reduced significantly from 2.12 ± 1.08 diopters to 0.48 ± 0.42 diopters (p = 0.01; Figure 1). Looking at the double-angle plot (Figure 2) and vector analysis, the centroid decreased from 1.37 ± 1.97 diopters at 90° preoperatively to 0.05 ± 0.64 diopters at 168° postoperatively (p = 0.03). In total, a residual refractive cylinder of 0.25 diopters or lower could be achieved in 42% of all patients, while in 58% the residual cylinder was 0.50 diopters or lower (Figure 1).

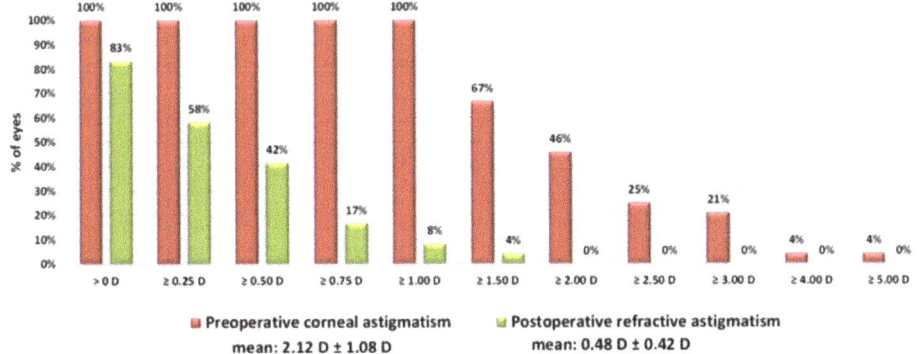

Figure 1. Cumulative histogram of the magnitudes of the preoperative corneal astigmatism and the postoperative refractive astigmatism at the corneal plane in the digital group (n = 24).

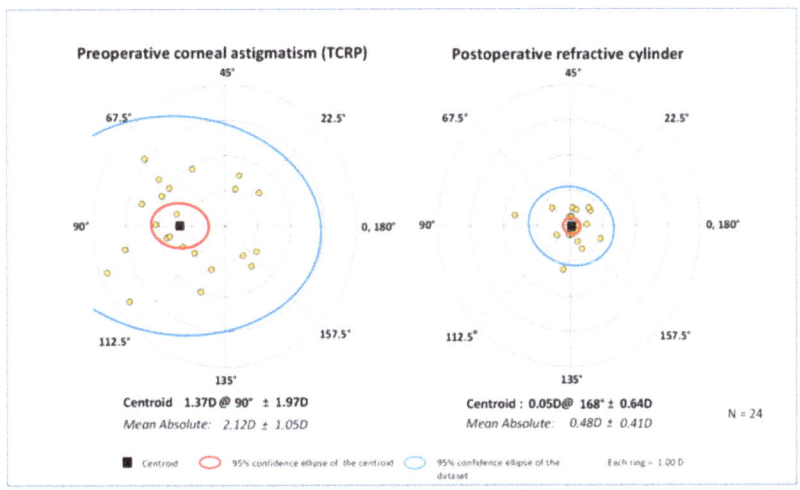

Figure 2. Double-angle plots of preoperative corneal astigmatism (TCRP) and postoperative refractive cylinder in the digital group (n = 24).

3.3. Prediction Error, Visual Outcome and Surgically Induced Astigmatism

The prediction error of spherical equivalent was 0.55 ± 0.43 diopters. Preoperative UDVA was 0.59 ± 0.18 logMAR and 0.4 ± 0.24 logMAR for CDVA. After 3 months, UDVA gained to 0.11 ± 0.09 logMAR and CDVA to 0.05 ± 0.08 logMAR. The mean vector or centroid of the actual postoperative surgically induced astigmatism was 0.21 diopters at 12°. Preoperatively, a SIA of 0.37 diopters at 2° was assumed. Thus, it was slightly overestimated. The SIA prediction error was 0.19 diopters at 9°.

3.4. Intraocular Lens Axis Misalignment

Intraocular lens axis was evaluated at the slit lamp. After three months, lens axis misalignment was $2.9 \pm 2.7°$. In total, 98% of all intraocular lenses were rotated less than 5 degrees. None of the intraocular lenses was re-rotated postoperatively.

4. Discussion

Based on our findings, the EQ Workplace within the FORUM platform, the onboard intraocular lens calculator Z CALC, as well as the CALLISTO eye and Z ALIGN digital tracking system offer a convenient and more efficient workflow for lens exchange surgery practice.

The preoperative time to identify the patient, check the biometric data, calculate the toric intraocular lens, and export the reference image for axis alignment was significantly less when the EQ Workplace within the FORUM platform was used. This might be due to the integrated intraocular lens calculator Z CALC and the automatic export of the reference image to the CALLISTO eye system in the operating room. Manually, biometric data must be double-checked on the IOLMaster 700 and the reference image must be transferred via an external storage device from the IOLMaster 700 to the CALLISTO eye system. Therefore, the software-based workflow approach is more efficient for surgeons preoperatively. During surgery, reference image matching and toric intraocular lens alignment is again easier and significantly faster using the digital image-guided approach, as the target axis does not have to be entered manually and the reference image import is basically one finger-tap on the touchscreen compared to the manual import from the USB stick. Thus, it offers surgeons a more comfortable experience prior to surgery. Furthermore, as the overall diagnostic and surgical time is significantly lower, rotation times can be minimized and lead to higher treatment numbers and a better economical outcome. In addition, transcription errors can be minimized when using a digital data transfer.

By increasing numbers of lens exchange surgeries on one day, surgeons and operators tend to mix up patient data and sides. According to a study by ophthalmologists in Israel, surgeons could only identify 73% of their surgical sides (left or right eye) correctly by knowing the patient's name. This error correlated with the actual number of surgeries performed on one day [11]. In the worst case, this might lead to the implantation of the wrong intraocular lens. Such an error could be minimized by using the EQ Workplace and FORUM platform cataract workflow, where calculated intraocular lenses are directly related to the surgical side and stored in the CALLISTO eye system on the surgical microscope.

The Z CALC intraocular lens calculator and its' featured intraocular lens calculation formula revealed a prediction error of 0.55 ± 0.43 diopters of spherical equivalent. More than 92% showed a residual cylinder of less than ± 1.00 diopters. Those results are in line with recent literature evaluating prediction errors of toric intraocular lenses using novel calculation formulas such as Barrett toric and Kane [12]. Furthermore, toric intraocular lens misalignment was low with a rotation of $2.9 \pm 2.7°$ and no need of any postoperative rotation in any of the subjects. Similar results comparing a manual-marking axis alignment to an image-guided approach corroborate our findings [13,14].

A limitation of our study might be the lack of a direct comparison between a fully manual approach of lens refractive surgery including intraoperative axis alignment by manual marking prior to surgery. This additional detail seemed obsolete as it was investigated before, as mentioned above [13,14]. The time for axis alignment in the digital group in the current study is significantly less statistically compared to the manual group, but, in our opinion, not of clinical relevance as the absolute difference barely accounts for 8 s. We consider those results a surgical bias.

Finally, one must take another issue into consideration: The system relies on a smart digital infrastructure that is costly, and in cases of technical malfunction might lead to severe delays and difficulties in daily lens exchange surgery routine.

To conclude, lens exchange surgery via the EQ Workplace within the FORUM platform is a safe and faster way to acquire and check data as well as to calculate intraocular lenses and align the lens axis intraoperatively compared to a manual approach. Thus, it guarantees a more efficient and economical workflow when performing cataract and lens refractive surgery.

Author Contributions: Conceptualization, B.S.B., S.K. and W.J.M.; methodology, W.J.M.; validation, S.K. and W.J.M.; formal analysis, B.S.B., S.K. and W.J.M.; investigation, M.S., S.G.P. and W.J.M.; resources, M.S., S.G.P. and W.J.M.; data curation, B.S.B., N.L., S.K.; writing—original draft preparation, B.S.B., S.K. and W.J.M.; writing—review and editing, M.S., N.L., S.G.P. and W.J.M.; visualization, S.K. and W.J.M.; supervision, M.S., N.L., S.G.P. and W.J.M.; funding acquisition, W.J.M. All authors have read and agreed to the published version of the manuscript.

Funding: This study 1890-21 (310) has been funded by an unrestricted research Grant from Carl Zeiss Meditec, Inc. The funders had no role in study design, data collection, analysis, decision to publish, or manuscript preparation.

Institutional Review Board Statement: The study was conducted in accordance with the Declaration of Helsinki and approved by the local institutional review board of the Ludwig Maximilian University (approval number: 19-731) for studies involving humans.

Informed Consent Statement: Informed consent was obtained from all subjects involved in the study.

Data Availability Statement: Not applicable.

Conflicts of Interest: Brunner BS: None. Luft N: Carl Zeiss Meditec AG, NIDEK Inc., Alcon AG. Priglinger SG: None. Shajari M: Alcon, Oculus, Carl Zeiss Meditec AG. Mayer WJ: Alcon AG, Carl Zeiss Meditec AG, Ziemer Ophthalmic Systems AG, DORC, Allergan, Teleon Surfical, Novartis AG, Bausch & Lomb, Heidelberg Engineering, Örtli, Staar Surgical, CSO, Humanoptics, Ophtec. Kassumeh S: None.

References

1. Łabuz, G.; Varadi, D.; Khoramnia, R.; Auffarth, G. Progressive-toric IOL design reduces residual astigmatism with increasing pupil size: A ray-tracing simulation based on corneal topography data. *Biomed. Opt. Express* **2021**, *12*, 1568–1576. [CrossRef] [PubMed]
2. Prasher, P.; Sandhu, J.S. Prevalence of corneal astigmatism before cataract surgery in Indian population. *Int. Ophthalmol.* **2017**, *37*, 683–689. [CrossRef] [PubMed]
3. De Bernardo, M.; Zeppa, L.; Cennamo, M.; Iaccarino, S.; Zeppa, L.; Rosa, N. Prevalence of corneal astigmatism before cataract surgery in Caucasian patients. *Eur. J. Ophthalmol.* **2014**, *24*, 494–500. [CrossRef] [PubMed]
4. Moulick, P.S.; Mohindra, V.K.; Gurunadh, V.S.; Patel, P.; Gupta, S.; Khan, M.A. A clinical study to evaluate the results after toric intraocular lens implantation in cases of corneal astigmatism. *Med. J. Armed Forces India* **2018**, *74*, 133–138. [CrossRef] [PubMed]
5. Khoramnia, R.; Auffarth, G.; Łabuz, G.; Pettit, G.; Suryakumar, R. Refractive Outcomes after Cataract Surgery. *Diagnostics* **2022**, *12*, 243. [CrossRef] [PubMed]
6. Fernández, J.; Rodríguez-Vallejo, M.; Burguera, N.; Salvestrini, P.; Garzón, N. Toric Intraocular Lens Results Considering Posterior Corneal Astigmatism with Online Calculators: Phacoemulsification vs. Femtosecond. *Optics* **2021**, *2*, 184–192. [CrossRef]
7. Fabian, E.; Wehner, W. Prediction Accuracy of Total Keratometry Compared to Standard Keratometry Using Different Intraocular Lens Power Formulas. *J. Refract. Surg.* **2019**, *35*, 362–368. [CrossRef] [PubMed]
8. Shi, Q.; Wang, G.Y.; Cheng, Y.H.; Pei, C. Comparison of IOL-Master 700 and IOL-Master 500 biometers in ocular biological parameters of adolescents. *Int. J. Ophthalmol.* **2021**, *14*, 1013–1017. [CrossRef] [PubMed]
9. Liu, B.; Kang, C.; Fang, F. Biometric Measurement of Anterior Segment: A Review. *Sensors* **2020**, *20*, 4285. [CrossRef] [PubMed]
10. Reinstein, D.Z.; Archer, T.J.; Srinivasan, S.; Mamalis, N.; Kohnen, T.; Dupps, W.J., Jr.; Randleman, J.B. Standard for reporting refractive outcomes of intraocular lens-based refractive surgery. *J. Cataract Refract. Surg.* **2017**, *43*, 435–439. [CrossRef] [PubMed]
11. Pikkel, D.; Sharabi-Nov, A.; Pikkel, J. It is the left eye, right? *Risk Manag. Healthc. Policy* **2014**, *7*, 77–80. [CrossRef] [PubMed]
12. Yang, S.; Byun, Y.S.; Kim, H.S.; Chung, S.H. Comparative Accuracy of Barrett Toric Calculator With and Without Posterior Corneal Astigmatism Measurements and the Kane Toric Formula. *Am. J. Ophthalmol.* **2021**, *231*, 48–57. [CrossRef] [PubMed]
13. Mayer, W.J.; Kreutzer, T.; Dirisamer, M.; Kern, C.; Kortuem, K.; Vounotrypidis, E.; Priglinger, S.; Kook, D. Comparison of visual outcomes, alignment accuracy, and surgical time between 2 methods of corneal marking for toric intraocular lens implantation. *J. Cataract Refract. Surg.* **2017**, *43*, 1281–1286. [CrossRef] [PubMed]
14. Barbera-Loustaunau, E.; Basanta, I.; Vazquez, J.; Duran, P.; Costa, M.; Counago, F.; Garzon, N.; Angel Sanchez-Tena, M. Time-efficiency assessment of guided toric intraocular lens cataract surgery: Pilot study. *J. Cataract Refract. Surg.* **2021**, *47*, 1535–1541. [CrossRef] [PubMed]

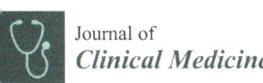

Article

A Comparison of Visual Quality and Contrast Sensitivity between Patients with Scleral-Fixated and In-Bag Intraocular Lenses

Yueh-Ling Chen [1,2], Christy Pu [3], Ken-Kuo Lin [1,2], Jiahn-Shing Lee [1,2], Laura Liu [1,2,*] and Chiun-Ho Hou [1,2,3,4,*]

1. Department of Ophthalmology, Chang Gung Memorial Hospital, Taoyuan 333, Taiwan; yuehling20@gmail.com (Y.-L.C.); d12093@cgmh.org.tw (K.-K.L.); leejsh@cgmh.org.tw (J.-S.L.)
2. Department of Medicine, School of Medicine, Chang Gung University, Taoyuan 333, Taiwan
3. Institute of Public Health, School of Medicine, National Yang Ming Chiao Tung University, Taipei 112, Taiwan; cypu@nycu.edu.tw
4. Department of Ophthalmology, National Taiwan University Hospital, Taipei 100, Taiwan
* Correspondence: laurajl@gmail.com (L.L.); chiunhohou@gmail.com (C.-H.H.); Tel.: +886-3-3281200 (ext. 8666) (C.-H.H.); Fax: +886-3-3287798 (C.-H.H.)

Abstract: Purpose: To analyze visual quality and contrast sensitivity in patients after intraocular lens (IOL) implantation with sutured scleral fixation. Setting: Chang Gung Memorial Hospital, Taoyuan, Taiwan. Design: Retrospective observational study. Methods: Data on the refractive outcome, visual acuity, and subjective visual symptoms in patients with scleral-fixated or in-bag IOL implantation were collected from September 2019 to March 2020. We also investigated patients' postoperative higher-order aberrations (HOAs) and dysphotopsia using a wavefront aberrometer and glaretester, respectively. The following values were compared: corrected distance visual acuity, spherical equivalent, root mean square values for aberrations, and contrast sensitivity. Results: A total of 23 eyes implanted with scleral-fixated IOL and 74 eyes with in-bag IOL were studied. The mean postoperative spherical equivalent and logarithm of the minimum angle of resolution after scleral fixation were -1.09 ± 3.32 D and 0.20 ± 0.17, respectively. The ocular HOAs were higher in the scleral-fixation group than in the in-bag group ($p = 0.001$). Contrast sensitivity was negatively associated with age, and it was similar between the two groups after controlling for the age effect. Conclusions: Ocular HOAs and refractive errors were higher in the scleral-fixation group than in the in-bag group. However, no significant difference was noted in contrast sensitivity between advanced scleral fixation and in-bag IOL implantation.

Keywords: visual quality; contrast sensitivity; scleral fixation; intraocular lens

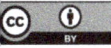

1. Introduction

Cataract surgery is the most common ocular surgery, with more than 20 million procedures performed worldwide [1]. Cataract surgery serves as both a visual restoration operation and refractive procedure [2]. Typically, the intraocular lens (IOL) is placed in a capsular bag. However, patients who experience posterior capsule rupture, zonular dialysis, dropped lens, or dislocated IOL during trauma or ocular surgery may receive alternative techniques such as anterior chamber, iris-fixated, or scleral-fixated IOLs [3].

The scleral-fixated IOL, first mentioned by Malbran [4] in 1986, has become a popular technique for patients with inadequate capsular support. The advantage of IOL scleral fixation over anterior chamber IOL implantation is the reduced risks of corneal endothelial loss, peripheral anterior synechiae, cystoid macular edema, and hyphema [5]. Although scleral-fixated IOL implantation has the problem of suture exposure, modified techniques can be applied to cover the suture ends with scleral pockets [6]. Another method is sutureless intrascleral-fixated IOL. A three-piece IOL is inserted into the anterior chamber, and the haptics are pulled out and positioned in the scleral tunnels. However, the complication of this technique includes intraoperative haptic breakdown [3].

Visual acuity can be maintained or improved with scleral fixation [7], but visual quality with regards to higher-order aberrations (HOAs) and contrast sensitivity remain issues. The IOL tilt and decentration after scleral fixation are greater than those after in-bag implantation [8]. IOL decentration can lead to dysphotopsia [9], and IOL tilt induces a considerable amount of ocular coma-like aberrations [10,11]. The appropriate positioning of an IOL is crucial to satisfactory visual quality following cataract surgery. However, the literature on dysphotopsia and contrast sensitivity after scleral-fixated IOL surgery is scant.

The purpose of this study was to compare the visual acuity, aberrometry, and glare disability of eyes treated with scleral fixation with those of eyes treated with standard cataract surgery.

2. Methods

2.1. Patients

This retrospective study comprised patients who underwent standard cataract surgery or transscleral fixation of the IOL. Inclusion criteria were as follows: patients with pseudophakia with in-bag or scleral-fixated IOLs, 20 years or older, no complications during IOL implantation, no ocular disorders such as severe non-proliferative diabetic retinopathy (NPDR) or PDR, corneal opacities or epithelial defects, severe macular degeneration or dystrophy, optic atrophy, amblyopia in the operated eye, or posterior capsule opacification after cataract surgery that could degrade visual quality. Indications for scleral fixation included aphakia and subluxation or dislocation of the crystalline lens or IOL. Only monofocal IOL implantation was studied because multifocal IOLs would have introduced a confounding effect with respect to dysphotopsia. We recruited patients between September 2019 and March 2020. Patients who could not undergo examination as a result of dementia or mental disorders were not included. All eyes had a minimum postoperative time of 1 month when the inflammation subsided without postoperative steroid use, corneal edema, or anterior chamber reaction, to ensure the wound and visual acuity were stable. We excluded patients with postoperative corrected distance visual acuity (CDVA) of more than 0.5 logarithm of the minimum angle of resolution (logMAR) because they could lose contrast sensitivity [12]. The study adhered to the tenets of the Declaration of Helsinki, and it was approved by the Institutional Review Board of Chang Gung Memorial Hospital, Taoyuan, Taiwan (Approval number: 2101220033). Written informed consent was waived because of the retrospective nature of the study.

2.2. Postoperative Ophthalmic Examinations

The CDVA was measured, and slit-lamp biomicroscopy, contrast sensitivity testing, pneumatic tonometry, indirect ophthalmoscopy, and aberrometry were performed. The postoperative CDVA was converted to logMAR values and compared between the scleral-fixation group and the in-bag group.

2.3. Contrast Sensitivity Test

Contrast sensitivity was evaluated with best refractive correction without pupil dilation using a CGT-2000 contrast glaretester (Takagi Seiko, Takaoka, Japan). Contrast sensitivity testing was performed under daytime (100 cd/m^2), twilight (10 cd/m^2), and nighttime (5 cd/m^2) luminance conditions with and without glare at a test distance of 5 m. The area under the log contrast sensitivity function (AULCSF) was calculated for statistical analysis [13].

Postoperative perceptive dysphotopsia was assessed using a questionnaire, with a point given for each category. Subjective photic phenomena, including glare, halo, starburst, and coma, were evaluated with a penlight held 1 m in front of the tested eye under mesopic conditions at the outpatient department. Symptoms were rated as 0 = none, 1 = mild, 2 = moderate, or 3 = severe. Additionally, this questionnaire was filled out by the nurse.

Higher mean scores indicated less satisfactory results. The mean score for each category was calculated and tested for significance.

2.4. Optical Aberrations

Wavefront measurements were postoperatively obtained using a refractive power and corneal analyzer (OPD-Scan III, NIDEK, Tokyo, Japan). This device used the fundamental principle of automatic retinoscopy, and it provided integrated corneal topography and wavefront measurement. The retina was scanned with a slit-shaped light beam, and the reflected light was captured by an array of rotating photodetectors over a 360° area. The aberrometer offered an aberration profile of the whole eye, and the root mean square values for aberrations, HOAs, tilt, coma, spherical aberrations, trefoil, and astigmatism were measured for statistical analysis. Wavefront maps were analyzed with a 3-mm pupil diameter up to the fourth-order Zernike coefficients. The pupil sizes were also measured by this wavefront aberrometer under mesopic condition.

2.5. Surgical Technique

Mydriasis was achieved preoperatively with 1% tropicamide eyedrops and 10% phenylephrine eyedrops. Sutured scleral fixation was performed by an experienced surgeon (LL), and phacoemulsification and in-bag IOL implantation were done by another (CHH). Scleral fixation was conducted using the four-point fixation technique described by Khan et al. [14], with some modifications. A 2.65-mm transparent corneal incision was made after retrobulbar anesthesia, and the IOL was loaded in the injector and injected into the anterior chamber. The two haptics were looped with a 10-0 polypropylene suture intraocularly at the nasal sclera 2 mm posterior to the limbus. The same step was repeated on the temporal side. Additional procedures such as vitrectomy and IOL exchange may have been performed at the time of scleral fixation. The standard phacoemulsification surgery was performed using the following procedures under topical anesthesia: clear corneal incision of 2.65 mm, continuous curvilinear capsulorrhexis with an approximate diameter of 5.0 mm, hydrodissection, phacoemulsification, irrigation and aspiration, and in-bag IOL implantation using an injector.

2.6. Statistical Analysis

All statistical analyses were performed using Stata, version 15 (StataCorp, College Station, TX, USA). Independent t tests were employed to compare the visual quality between the two groups. Generalized estimate equation method (GEE) was performed to identify factors affecting contrast sensitivity, which was set as the dependent variable (AULCSF). The following parameters were included as explanatory variables: age, sex, pupil size, surgical technique (scleral fixation or in-bag IOL implantation), IOL type (spherical, aspheric, or toric), logMAR, and ocular aberrations. Another GEE was conducted to determine the factors affecting subjective dysphotopsia (glare, halo, starburst, and coma), with the same aforementioned explanatory variables. A p value of less than 0.05 was considered statistically significant.

3. Results

This study comprised 100 eyes from 70 patients. Three eyes from three patients were excluded because the CDVA was greater than 0.5 logMAR. A total of 97 eyes from 67 patients were analyzed, of which 23 eyes underwent sutured scleral fixation, with a mean patient age of 58.13 years (range 36–79 years), and 74 eyes underwent in-bag IOL implantation, with a mean patient age of 69.76 years (range 46–96 years). A total of 15 eyes (20.27%) of 10 patients had diabetes mellitus in the in-bag group, while 6 eyes (26.09%) of 5 patients were affected in the scleral-fixated group. One patient in the in-bag group had Sjogren's syndrome. The mean spherical equivalent was -1.09 ± 3.32 D in the scleral-fixation group and -0.23 ± 0.75 D in the in-bag group. The CDVA of the in-bag group was slightly better (mean logMAR 0.11 vs. 0.20). Statistically significant differences were observed between the two groups in terms of age, sex, IOL type, CDVA, and spherical equivalent (Table 1). Although 33 eyes (34%) were followed within 3 months after the surgery, the mean CDVA could reach 0.16 logMAR. In the scleral-fixation group, 14 eyes had IOL subluxation or dislocation; 4 eyes had lens dislocation and 5 had aphakia following complications with cataract extraction. The majority of sutured IOLs in the scleral-fixated group (56.52%) received Akreos Adapt Advanced Optics lenses (Bausch + Lomb, Laval, QC, Canada).

Table 1. Demographics and visual outcomes of eyes following in-bag and scleral-fixated intraocular lens implantation.

Characteristics	In-Bag (n = 74)	Scleral Fixation (n = 23)	p Value
Age in years, mean ± SD (range)	69.76 ± 9.58 (46–96)	58.13 ± 12.81 (36–79)	<0.001 *
Male sex, No. (male %)	24 (32.43)	10 (43.48)	0.038 *
Laterality, No.			0.509
OD (%)	36 (48.65)	13 (56.52)	
OS (%)	38 (51.35)	10 (43.48)	
IOL type, No.			0.003 *
Spherical (%)	19 (25.68)	9 (39.13)	
Aspheric (%)	28 (37.84)	14 (60.87)	
Toric (%)	27 (36.48)	0 (0)	
Postop in months, mean ± SD (range)	19.88 ± 30.09 (1–132)	16.22 ± 19.27 (1–60)	0.585
Pupil size (mm ± SD)	4.81 ± 1.02	4.66 ± 0.99	0.526
CDVA (logMAR ± SD)	0.11 ± 0.14	0.20 ± 0.17	0.015 *
SE, mean ± SD	−0.23 ± 0.75	−1.09 ± 3.32	0.0385 *
Astigmatism, mean ± SD	−0.81 ± 0.58	−1.11 ± 0.87	0.0654

CDVA = corrected distance visual acuity; IOL = intraocular lens; logMAR = logarithm of the minimum angle of resolution; OD = right eye; OS = left eye; SD = standard deviation; SE = spherical equivalent; * $p < 0.05$.

The postoperative wavefront data including ocular, internal, and corneal aberrations for both groups are listed in Table 2. Ocular aberrations differed markedly from corneal aberrations between the scleral-fixation and the in-bag group in terms of overall aberrations, HOAs, tilt, coma, trefoil, and astigmatism, with the exception of spherical aberrations.

Table 2. Postoperative ocular, corneal, and internal aberrations for 3-mm pupil diameters in eyes following in-bag and scleral-fixated intraocular lens implantation.

	In-Bag (n = 74)	Scleral Fixation (n = 23)	p Value
Ocular			
Aberrations [a] (μm ± SD)	0.387 ± 0.194	0.785 ± 0.667	<0.001 *
HOAs (μm ± SD)	0.145 ± 0.070	0.255 ± 0.241	0.001 *
Tilt (μm ± SD)	0.103 ± 0.064	0.187 ± 0.203	0.003 *
Trefoil (μm ± SD)	0.121 ± 0.076	0.209 ± 0.189	0.002 *
Coma (μm ± SD)	0.035 ± 0.024	0.058 ± 0.053	0.004 *
Astigmatism [b] (μm ± SD)	0.434 ± 0.211	0.704 ± 0.553	0.001 *
Spherical aberration (μm ± SD)	0.016 ± 0.013	0.022 ± 0.020	0.059
Corneal			
Aberrations [a] (μm ± SD)	0.377 ± 0.183	0.432 ± 0.194	0.213
HOAs (μm ± SD)	0.112 ± 0.049	0.146 ± 0.084	0.019 *
Tilt (μm ± SD)	0.133 ± 0.102	0.167 ± 0.148	0.208
Trefoil (μm ± SD)	0.074 ± 0.042	0.102 ± 0.066	0.017 *
Coma (μm ± SD)	0.056 ± 0.038	0.065 ± 0.060	0.355
Astigmatism [b] (μm ± SD)	1.201 ± 0.828	1.340 ± 0.739	0.473
Spherical aberration (μm ± SD)	0.025 ± 0.024	0.035 ± 0.030	0.094
Internal			
Aberrations [a] (μm ± SD)	0.404 ± 0.204	0.714 ± 0.683	0.001 *
HOAs (μm ± SD)	0.130 ± 0.066	0.209 ± 0.234	0.011 *
Tilt (μm ± SD)	0.138 ± 0.110	0.178 ± 0.177	0.198
Trefoil (μm ± SD)	0.086 ± 0.061	0.151 ± 0.173	0.007 *
Coma (μm ± SD)	0.051 ± 0.041	0.053 ± 0.037	0.830
Astigmatism [b] (μm ± SD)	0.858 ± 0.685	1.340 ± 1.815	0.060
Spherical aberration (μm ± SD)	0.025 ± 0.024	0.035 ± 0.030	0.094

HOAs = higher-order aberrations; * $p < 0.05$; [a] lower and higher-order aberrations included; [b] astigmatism and secondary astigmatism included.

In terms of contrast sensitivity testing, the in-bag group performed better under daytime luminance conditions with or without glare interference but similar to those in the scleral-fixation group under twilight or night conditions (Table 3). For the in-bag group and scleral-fixation group, 53 (71.62%) and 11 eyes (47.83%) were tested for perceptive dysphotopsia, respectively. The mean questionnaire scores for subjective dysphotopsia under mesopic conditions with glare showed no significant differences between the two groups. Symptoms of glare, halo, coma, and starburst were similar in both groups ($p > 0.5$).

Table 3. Postoperative contrast sensitivity of eyes following in-bag and scleral-fixated intraocular lens implantation.

(AULCSF ± SD)	In-Bag ($n = 74$)	Scleral Fixation ($n = 23$)	p Value
Day (100 cd/m^2)			
Glare off	1.345 ± 0.395	1.073 ± 0.549	0.011 *
Glare on	1.314 ± 0.333	1.065 ± 0.521	0.008 *
Twilight (10 cd/m^2)			
Glare off	1.179 ± 0.317	1.046 ± 0.434	0.114
Glare on	1.060 ± 0.356	0.887 ± 0.479	0.065
Night (5 cd/m^2)			
Glare off	1.085 ± 0.316	0.972 ± 0.371	0.157
Glare on	0.783 ± 0.359	0.658 ± 0.443	0.173

AULCSF = area under the log contrast sensitivity function; * $p < 0.05$.

The results of GEE for contrast sensitivity are described in Figure 1 and Table 4. Age had significantly negative effects on contrast sensitivity under photopic and mesopic conditions, and the surgical technique (in-bag and scleral fixation) did not affect the results of contrast sensitivity after controlling for the age effect. LogMAR and ocular aberrations had significantly negative effects on contrast sensitivity under every luminance condition with or without glare interference. No significant variable was determined in the GEE for dysphotopsia.

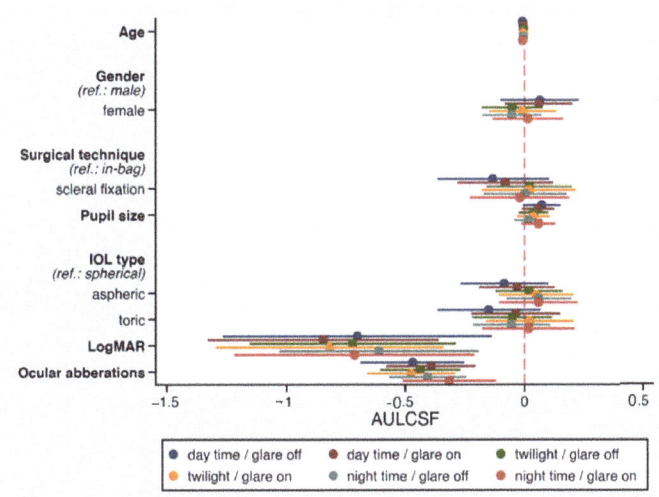

Figure 1. Forest plot depicts the coefficient of each factor and its 95% confidence interval (CI) in a multiple regression analysis for factors associated with contrast sensitivity. The x-axis represents the reference line (dashed), the value of coefficient (dot), and 95% CI (strip). AULCSF = area under the log contrast sensitivity function; IOL = intraocular lens; LogMAR = logarithm of the minimum angle of resolution.

Table 4. Multivariate generalized estimating equation (GEE) analysis of contrast sensitivity under every luminance condition with or without glare interference.

Variables		Day Time Glare off	Day Time Glare on	Twilight Glare off	Twilight Glare on	Night Time Glare off	Night Time Glare on
		β (SE)	β (SE)	β (SE)	β (SE)	β (SE)	β (SE)
Age		−0.008 (0.004) *	−0.008 (0.004) *	−0.005 (0.003)	−0.007 (0.004)	−0.007 (0.003) *	−0.009 (0.004) *
Gender		0.080 (0.082)	0.095 (0.076)	−0.027 (0.070)	0.013 (0.073)	−0.027 (0.069)	0.030 (0.077)
Surgical technique		−0.127 (0.113)	−0.145 (0.097)	−0.012 (0.085)	−0.014 (0.096)	−0.039 (0.082)	−0.053 (0.102)
Pupil size		0.069 (0.039)	0.035 (0.034)	0.007 (0.029)	0.014 (0.033)	−0.024 (0.028)	0.032 (0.035)
IOL type	Aspheric	−0.077 (0.091)	−0.007 (0.082)	0.097 (0.074)	0.077 (0.080)	0.122 (0.072)	0.075 (0.084)
	Toric	−0.126 (0.107)	−0.015 (0.093)	0.036 (0.081)	0.059 (0.092)	0.040 (0.078)	0.042 (0.097)
LogMAR		−0.698 (0.277) *	−0.700 (0.235) **	−0.590 (0.200) ***	−0.776 (0.234) **	−0.406 (0.191) **	−0.677 (0.248) *
Ocular aberrations		−0.460 (0.106) ***	−0.387 (0.090) ***	−0.417 (0.078) ***	−0.458 (0.090) ***	−0.405 (0.075) ***	−0.333 (0.095) ***

IOL = intraocular lens; logMAR = logarithm of the minimum angle of resolution; SE = standard error; * $p < 0.05$, ** $p < 0.01$; *** $p < 0.001$.

4. Discussion

This study demonstrated that the mean CDVA, spherical equivalent, and ocular HOAs were significantly better in the in-bag group than in the scleral-fixation group. However, in the contrast sensitivity test, no difference was noted between the groups except under photopic conditions, which was compatible with the result of the subjective dysphotopsia questionnaire. The factors related to low-contrast sensitivity were age, logMAR, and ocular aberrations.

Mimura et al. [15] reported that the mean spherical equivalent was −1.16 ± 2.28 D for transscleral-fixated IOL implantation at 2 years, and Mizuno et al. [16] indicated that the mean postoperative CDVA in the logMAR at 1 month was 0.25 ± 0.41. Both results were similar to those of our study. Huang et al. [17] determined that IOL scleral fixation induced an average 1.66 D myopic shift, which may be caused by the more anterior placement of the scleral-fixated IOLs [16]. Hayashi et al. [8] demonstrated that anterior chamber depth with sutured IOLs was shallower than that with in-bag IOLs, which caused a significant myopic shift. Other studies [18–21] have also reported an increase in spherical equivalent in those who underwent IOL scleral fixation.

Most of our patients who received transscleral IOL fixation were men, and they were much younger than those who underwent in-bag IOL implantation. The main reason for scleral fixation was trauma experienced during labor work, and the majority of laborers were men. One study [15] with a 12-year follow-up noted that the mean patient age after scleral fixation was 61.7 years, and another study [10] recorded more men in their scleral-fixation group than in the in-bag group (44.4% vs. 41%), which was similar to our study.

Ocular coma aberration was significantly greater in the scleral-fixation group than in the in-bag group. A study [10] indicated that IOL tilt correlated with ocular coma-like aberrations. Therefore, an increase in ocular coma aberrations in the scleral-fixation group in our study suggests the contribution of an IOL tilt. Ocular trefoil aberration was also greater after scleral fixation. Torii et al. [22] noted the same results and reported that postoperative ocular, corneal, and internal trefoil-like aberrations were significantly greater in their scleral-fixation group than in the intracapsular group. Spherical aberration was correlated with the implanted IOL type, and aspheric IOLs were associated with lower spherical aberrations than spherical IOLs. Our results demonstrated that the percentage of aspheric IOLs, including those that were toric, in the scleral-fixation group was comparable to that in the in-bag group (74.32% vs. 60.87%, $p = 0.21$), indicating no difference in ocular spherical aberration between the two groups.

In this study, we observed that patients with scleral-fixated IOLs had worse contrast sensitivity only under photopic conditions, which may be attributable to poor visual acuity and more ocular aberrations in this group. Additionally, visual acuity may predict contrast sensitivity. Rubin et al. [23] reported a linear regression with a correlation coefficient of −0.56 for the logMAR and contrast sensitivity in patients with cataracts. Another study [24] demonstrated consistent results, with a significant correlation between the logMAR and contrast sensitivity ($r = -0.55$). Contrast sensitivity was also affected by ocular aberrations in this study. Many studies [25,26] have reported that deteriorated contrast sensitivity is related to increased HOAs in eyes that underwent keratorefractive surgery. For cataract surgery, however, no studies have indicated such results. Our result suggested that an increase in ocular aberrations contributed to the loss of contrast sensitivity in pseudophakic eyes, which has never before been published. Research into contrast sensitivity in patients with scleral-fixated IOLs was scarce. Gao et al. [27] concluded that IOL decentration and a tilt less than 0.5 mm and 5°, respectively, did not affect postoperative contrast sensitivity under dim light conditions. The results of perceptive dysphotopsia tested in our study also indicated no significant difference between these two groups under mesopic conditions. In the multivariate regression, surgical technique did not significantly affect the extent of subjective glare disability.

Most patients in the scleral-fixation group received Akreos IOLs four-point fixation. Compared with traditional two-point scleral fixation, this technique has a low risk of IOL tilt and decentration. In addition, cystoid macular edema and glaucoma were less commonly observed with four-point fixation [28]. With regard to other complications after suture-fixated IOL procedures, only one suture exposure was noted in our study, which was markedly low compared with a report indicating a 6–27% probability of suture-related complications in transscleral-sutured IOL surgery [5].

Our study had several limitations. First, the sample size of the scleral-fixation group was not large, but the subjective and the objective refraction were both consistent with those of other studies. Second, in this study, we could not evaluate the preoperative visual function because many of our patients were referred from other medical facilities for IOL fixation, and we could not assess the extent of visual improvement following surgery in the scleral fixation group. The causes for inferior CDVA in scleral fixation group could be our fixation method or prior insults, such as trauma or a complication of cataract surgery. This is intrinsic, and it is not possible to differentiate. However, our result showed that with an advanced scleral fixation technique, patients subjectively did not suffer from worse contrast sensitivity than patients with in-bag IOL implantation. Third, several different IOL types were used in our study, providing different spherical aberrations of IOLs, which affected ocular spherical aberrations [2,29–31]. However, the percentage of spherical or aspheric IOLs in these two groups was similar, as were the ocular and the internal spherical aberrations. In our multivariate generalized estimating equation analysis, the IOL type (spherical, aspheric, or toric) had no significant effect on contrast sensitivity. Fourth, the patients in the scleral-fixated group were younger than those in the in-bag group, and age was reported to have a negative effect on contrast sensitivity [32,33]. Our result also demonstrated that patients with older age were associated with worse contrast sensitivity. However, after controlling for the age effect, the surgical technique (in-bag and scleral fixation) did not affect the results of contrast sensitivity. Finally, instead of using commercially available dysphotopsia questionnaires [34], we utilized a newly designed method of evaluating dysphotopsia under simulated nighttime luminance. The strength of our study was the simultaneous investigation of objective contrast sensitivity and subjective glare disability following transscleral-sutured IOLs procedures, both of which provided consistent results.

In summary, our study demonstrated that although the logMAR, spherical equivalent, and higher-order aberrations were greater following scleral fixation, there was no significant difference between scleral-fixated IOLs and in-bag IOL implantation in terms of the visual quality and the contrast sensitivity under mesopic conditions. The age, logMAR, and ocular aberrations had negative effects on contrast sensitivity in patients with pseudophakia under different luminance conditions. It is noteworthy that perceptive dysphotopsia under a dim light was similar between these two groups, which means the patients' satisfaction was comparable, and it is as convincing as the objective measurements when evaluating visual quality. In addition, our study suggested that careful manipulation by a well-experienced surgeon could provide satisfactory outcomes in patients who received transscleral-sutured IOLs with four-point fixation. However, refinement of suturing techniques in sclera fixation is still required to reduce ocular aberrations and to preserve contrast sensitivity under daylight conditions. Further studies should include a larger sample size, sutureless technique, and matched case-control study design, such as age, sex, and visual outcome, to deepen our understanding of the visual quality of IOL scleral fixation.

Author Contributions: Conceptualization, K.-K.L., J.-S.L. and C.-H.H.; Data curation, Y.-L.C., L.L. and C.-H.H.; Formal analysis, Y.-L.C., C.P. and C.-H.H.; Investigation, L.L. and C.-H.H.; Methodology C.P., L.L. and C.-H.H.; Project administration, Y.-L.C. and C.P.; Resources, K.-K.L., J.-S.L., L.L. and C.-H.H.; Software, C.P.; Supervision, K.-K.L. and J.-S.L.; Validation, K.-K.L. and J.-S.L.; Visualization Y.-L.C. and C.P.; Writing—original draft, Y.-L.C.; Writing—review & editing, L.L. and C.-H.H. All authors have read and agreed to the published version of the manuscript.

Funding: This research received no external funding.

Institutional Review Board Statement: The study adhered to the tenets of the Declaration of Helsinki, and it was approved by the Institutional Review Board of Chang Gung Memorial Hospital Taoyuan, Taiwan (Approval number: 2101220033).

Informed Consent Statement: Written informed consent was waived because of the retrospective nature of the study.

Data Availability Statement: Not applicable.

Conflicts of Interest: The authors declare no conflict of interest.

References

1. Lindstrom, R. Thoughts on cataract surgery: 2015. *Rev. Ophthalmol.* **2015**. Available online: http://www.reviewofophthalmology.com/content/t/surgical_education/c/53422 (accessed on 28 May 2021).
2. Jirásková, N. Optical Aberrations and Contrast Sensitivity of Spherical and Aspheric Intraocular Lenses—A Prospective Comparative Clinical Study. *J. Clin. Exp. Ophthalmol.* **2012**, *3*, 9. [CrossRef]
3. Matsuki, N.; Inoue, M.; Itoh, Y.; Nagamoto, T.; Hirakata, A. Changes in higher-order aberrations of intraocular lenses with intrascleral fixation. *Br. J. Ophthalmol.* **2015**, *99*, 1732–1738. [CrossRef]
4. Malbran, E.S.; Malbran, E., Jr.; Negri, I. Lens guide suture for transport and fixation in secondary IOL implantation after intracapsular extraction. *Int. Ophthalmol.* **1986**, *9*, 151–160. [CrossRef] [PubMed]
5. Luk, A.S.W.; Young, A.L.; Cheng, L.L. Long-term outcome of scleral-fixated intraocular lens implantation. *Br. J. Ophthalmol.* **2013**, *97*, 1308–1311. [CrossRef]
6. Long, C.; Wei, Y.; Yuan, Z.; Zhang, Z.; Lin, X.; Liu, B. Modified technique for transscleral fixation of posterior chamber intraocular lenses. *BMC Ophthalmol.* **2015**, *15*, 127. [CrossRef] [PubMed]
7. Por, Y.M.; Lavin, M.J. Techniques of intraocular lens suspension in the absence of capsular/zonular support. *Surv. Ophthalmol.* **2005**, *50*, 429–462. [CrossRef]
8. Hayashi, K.; Hayashi, H.; Nakao, F.; Hayashi, F. Intraocular lens tilt and decentration, anterior chamber depth, and refractive error after trans-scleral suture fixation surgery. *Ophthalmology* **1999**, *106*, 878–882. [CrossRef]
9. Kozaki, J.; Tanilhara, H.; Yasuda, A.; Nagata, M. Tilt and decentration of the implanted posterior chamber intraocular lens. *J. Cataract. Refract. Surg.* **1991**, *17*, 592–595. [CrossRef]
10. Oshika, T.; Sugita, G.; Miyata, K.; Tokunaga, T.; Samejima, T.; Okamoto, C.; Ishii, Y. Influence of tilt and decentration of scleral-sutured intraocular lens on ocular higher-order wavefront aberration. *Br. J. Ophthalmol.* **2007**, *91*, 185–188. [CrossRef]
11. Taketani, F.; Matuura, T.; Yukawa, E.; Hara, Y. Influence of intraocular lens tilt and decentration on wavefront aberrations. *J. Cataract Refract. Surg.* **2004**, *30*, 2158–2162. [CrossRef] [PubMed]
12. Elliott, D.B.; Gilchrist, J.; Whitaker, D. Contrast sensitivity and glare sensitivity changes with three types of cataract morphology: Are these techniques necessary in a clinical evaluation of cataract? *Ophthalmic Physiol. Opt.* **1989**, *9*, 25–30. [CrossRef] [PubMed]
13. Applegate, R.A.; Howland, H.C.; Sharp, R.P.; Cottingham, A.J.; Yee, R.W. Corneal aberrations and visual performance after radial keratotomy. *J. Retract. Surg.* **1998**, *14*, 397–4071. [CrossRef] [PubMed]
14. Khan, M.A.; Rahimy, E.; Gupta, O.P.; Hsu, J. Combined 27-Gauge Pars Plana Vitrectomy and Scleral Fixation of an Akreos AO60 Intraocular Lens Using Gore-Tex Suture. *Retina* **2016**, *36*, 1602–1604. [CrossRef]
15. Mimura, T.; Amano, S.; Sugiura, T.; Funatsu, H.; Yamagami, S.; Araie, M.; Eguchi, S. Refractive change after transscleral fixation of posterior chamber intraocular lenses in the absence of capsular support. *Acta Ophthalmol. Scand.* **2004**, *82*, 544–546. [CrossRef]
16. Mizuno, Y.; Sugimoto, Y. A comparative study of transscleral suture-fixated and scleral-fixated intraocular lens implantation. *Int. Ophthalmol.* **2019**, *39*, 839–845. [CrossRef]

7. Huang, Y.-C.; Tseng, C.-C.; Lin, C.-P. Myopic shift of sulcus suture-fixated posterior chamber intraocular lenses. *Taiwan J. Ophthalmol.* **2013**, *3*, 95–97. [CrossRef]
8. Bayramlar, H.; Hepsen, I.F.; Yilmaz, H. Myopic shift from the predicted refraction after sulcus fixation of PMMA posterior chamber intraocular lenses. *Can. J. Ophthalmol.* **2006**, *41*, 78–82. [CrossRef]
9. Ma, D.J.; Choi, H.J.; Kim, M.K.; Wee, W.R. Clinical comparison of ciliary sulcus and pars plana locations for posterior chamber intraocular lens transscleral fixation. *J. Cataract. Refract. Surg.* **2011**, *37*, 1439–1446. [CrossRef]
10. Olsen, T. Sources of error in intraocular lens power calculation. *J. Cataract. Refract. Surg.* **1992**, *18*, 125–129. [CrossRef]
11. Suto, C.; Hori, S.; Fukuyama, E.; Akura, J. Adjusting intraocular lens power for sulcus fixation. *J. Cataract. Refract. Surg.* **2003**, *29*, 1913–1917. [CrossRef]
12. Torii, T.; Tamaoki, A.; Kojima, T.; Matsuda, T.; Kaga, T.; Ichikawa, K. Comparison of Clinical Outcomes Between Intracapsular Implantation and Intrascleral Fixation Using the Same Model of Intraocular Lens. *Clin. Ophthalmol.* **2020**, *14*, 3965–3974. [CrossRef] [PubMed]
13. Rubin, G.S.; Adamsons, I.A.; Stark, W.J. Comparison of acuity, contrast sensitivity, and disability glare before and after cataract surgery. *Arch. Ophthalmol.* **1993**, *111*, 56–61. [CrossRef] [PubMed]
14. Elliott, D.B.; Hurst, M.A. Simple clinical techniques to evaluate visual function in patients with early cataract. *Optom. Vis. Sci.* **1990**, *67*, 822–825. [CrossRef] [PubMed]
15. Tanabe, T.; Miyata, K.; Samejima, T.; Hirohara, Y.; Mihashi, T.; Oshika, T. Influence of wavefront aberration and corneal subepithelial haze on low-contrast visual acuity after photorefractive keratectomy. *Am. J. Ophthalmol.* **2004**, *138*, 620–624. [CrossRef]
16. Yamane, N.; Miyata, K.; Samejima, T.; Hiraoka, T.; Kiuchi, T.; Okamoto, F.; Hirohara, Y.; Mihashi, T.; Oshika, T. Ocular higher-order aberrations and contrast sensitivity after conventional laser in situ keratomileusis. *Investig. Ophthalmol. Vis. Sci.* **2004**, *45*, 3986–3990. [CrossRef]
17. Gao, S.; Qin, T.; Wang, S.; Lu, Y. Sulcus Fixation of Foldable Intraocular Lenses Guided by Ultrasound Biomicroscopy. *J. Ophthalmol.* **2015**, *2015*, 520418. [CrossRef]
18. Fass, O.N.; Herman, W.K. Four-point suture scleral fixation of a hydrophilic acrylic IOL in aphakic eyes with insufficient capsule support. *J. Cataract. Refract. Surg.* **2010**, *36*, 991–996. [CrossRef]
19. Casprini, F.; Balestrazzi, A.; Tosi, G.M.; Miracco, F.; Martone, G.; Cevenini, G.; Caporossi, A. Glare disability and spherical aberration with five foldable intraocular lenses: A prospective randomized study. *Acta Ophthalmol. Scand.* **2005**, *83*, 20–25. [CrossRef]
20. Kim, S.W.; Ahn, H.; Kim, E.K.; Kim, T.I. Comparison of higher order aberrations in eyes with aspherical or spherical intraocular lenses. *Eye* **2008**, *22*, 1493–1498. [CrossRef]
21. Ang, R.T.; Martinez, G.A.; Caguioa, J.B.; Reyes, K.B. Comparison in the quality of vision and spherical aberration between spherical and aspheric intraocular lenses. *Philipp. J. Ophthalmol.* **2008**, *33*, 9.
22. Arundale, K. An investigation into the variation of human contrast sensitivity with age and ocular pathology. *Br. J. Ophthalmol.* **1978**, *62*, 213–215. [CrossRef] [PubMed]
23. Hohberger, B.; Laemmer, R.; Adler, W.; Juenemann, A.G.; Horn, F.K. Measuring contrast sensitivity in normal subjects with OPTEC 6500: Influence of age and glare. *Graefe's Arch. Clin. Exp. Ophthalmol.* **2007**, *245*, 1805–1814. [CrossRef] [PubMed]
24. Grzybowski, A.; Kanclerz, P.; Muzyka-Woźniak, M. Methods for evaluating quality of life and vision in patients undergoing lens refractive surgery. *Graefe's Arch. Clin. Exp. Ophthalmol.* **2019**, *257*, 1091–1099. [CrossRef]

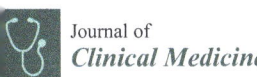

Reply

Reply to Cione et al. Comment on "Iida et al. Development of a New Method for Calculating Intraocular Lens Power after Myopic Laser In Situ Keratomileusis by Combining the Anterior–Posterior Ratio of the Corneal Radius of the Curvature with the Double-K Method. *J. Clin. Med.* 2022, 11, 522"

Yoshihiko Iida [1,*], Kimiya Shimizu [2] and Nobuyuki Shoji [1]

[1] Department of Ophthalmology, Kitasato University School of Medicine, Sagamihara 252-0374, Japan; nshoji@kitasato-u.ac.jp
[2] Eye Center, Sanno Hospital, Tokyo 107-0052, Japan; kimiyas@iuhw.ac.jp
* Correspondence: yiida@kitasato-u.ac.jp

We appreciate the insightful comments [1] on our article [2]. We reply as follows:

(1) We agree with their opinion that the paper by Rosa et al., where a formula to estimate keratometry (K) before refractive surgery (Kpre) based on the postoperative posterior corneal power was proposed [3], is important for this topic and thus should have been cited in this article.

(2) The corneal refractive power used in the SRK/T formula is optimized to the keratometric value, which estimates the total corneal refractive power from the anterior surface of the cornea. The ISS method is a double-K method based on the SRK/T formula using the K value with the IOL master and the axial length of the eye, and it is not appropriate to directly input the Pentacam measurements as the Kpost [4]. Therefore, the ISS method uses the IOL Master measurements to calculate IOL power using the Double-K method, determines the C-factor based on the correlation between the refractive error of Double-K method and the A-P ratio derived from Pentacam, and adjusts the target refraction value. The Pentacam measurements are only used to determine the A-P ratio of corneal curvature, and do not correspond to the point made by Cione et al. that data derived from different machines cannot be used interchangeably. Incidentally, there are other instruments besides the Pentacam that can measure and calculate the anterior–posterior corneal curvature ratio, including anterior segment OCT, but since the measurement principle is different, we believe that the anterior–posterior corneal curvature ratio measured with anterior segment OCT cannot be used in the ISS method without modification. Therefore, it should be noted that the calculation of the A-P ratio is not compatible between different models. If the A-P ratio measured by anterior segment OCT is to be used, it is necessary to calculate the C-factor from the correlation between the A-P ratio measured by anterior segment OCT and the refractive error of the Double-K method.

(3) Our study was designed to compare the ISS method with other IOL calculation methods commonly used for cataract surgery in the post-LASIK eye, primarily those included in the American Society of Cataract and Refractive Surgery calculator, rather than an exhaustive comparison of all methods. We hope to compare other IOL power calculations in the future, including ALMA [5], which is not included in the ASCRS calculator.

(4) Regarding the evaluation of PE, as has been pointed out, the conversion from IOL PE to PE is an estimate, and there may be differences in the amount of PE change per 1 D depending on the IOL degree. In the present study, the mean IOL power was 20.63 ± 2.20 D (15.0–24.0 D), and many cases used a power around 20.0 D, which may have caused errors in the IOL PE to PE conversion but had relatively little effect on the results. Furthermore, the optical design of IOLs differs depending on the type of IOL, which may affect the

amount of change, but only one type of IOL was used in this study, and the influence of the type of IOL on the error was eliminated. However, this is a limitation of this evaluation method, as indicated by Cione et al.

(5) Although the IOL power calculation analysis for normal eyes requires a process of optimizing the IOL constant for the data set to achieve a mean error (ME) of 0, deriving an optimized IOL constant for a special case such as post-LASIK eyes in clinical practice is not an exact process or applicable to future cases; some have suggested that it is inappropriate because it is not considered possible [6]. In addition, the number of cases of atypical eyes is small, and it is difficult to optimize the IOL constants. What is clinically required is a formula that can be used with the same constants as for normal eyes and still provide accurate results. Therefore, in this study, IOL power calculations were performed using standard IOL constants optimized for normal eyes, and no further optimization of the data set of IOL constants was performed. The ISS method has the advantage of using the A constant of the SRK/T formula, which is optimized for normal eyes.

(6) The papers published in the past 10 years indicate that it is advisable to publish studies that include a sample size of about 200 eyes for normal eyes and at least 50 eyes for atypical eyes, such as after refractive surgery [7]. The cases in the current study were limited to one eye per patient and one type of IOL, which we hope will reduce the possibility of statistical error. It should be added that all of the objective eyes in this study were limited to cases in which 20/20 or better visual acuity was achieved, which does not mean that the accuracy of the postoperative refractive error is insufficient.

As for the statistics, data were verified for non-normality using the Kolmogorov-Smirnov test. The percentages of eyes within ±0.25 D, ±0.50 D, and ±1.00 D of PE were compared using Fisher's exact test and Bonferroni correction, following the methods used in previous reports [8,9].

We compared the percentage of eyes within ±0.25, ±0.50 and ±1.00 D of PE by Cochran's Q test [7], as suggested by Cione et al. The percentages of eyes within ±0.25 D, ±0.50 D, and ±1.00 D of PE were significantly different ($p < 0.0001$, $p < 0.0001$, $p = 0.006$) respectively. Furthermore, the comparison between formulas was analyzed by the McNemar test with Bonferroni correction, and the ISS method was significantly better than the Potvin–Hill Pentacam method at ±0.25 D ($p = 0.015$). At ±0.50 D, the ISS method was better than the Potvin–Hill Pentacam method ($p = 0.044$) and significantly better than the Haigis-L formula ($p = 0.044$), and at ±1.00 D, the Cochran Q test showed a significant difference, but no significant difference could be detected in the comparison between each formula.

We would like to add a comment about the evaluation of the median absolute value of error (MedAE), as suggested by Cione et al. The Friedman test with a post hoc test (Bonferroni multiple test) showed that the ISS method was significantly different from all formulas ($p < 0.0001$ for all) except the Barrett True-K formula; the Shammas No-history method and the Haigis-L formula were significantly different from the Potvin–Hill Pentacam method ($p = 0.001$, $p = 0.0001$); and the Barrett True-K formula was significantly different from the Shammas No-history method and the Potvin-Hill Pentacam method ($p = 0.019$, $p < 0.0001$).

As mentioned above, although results with additional statistical analysis are also shown, the predictability of the ISS method was equal to or better than several other formulas. In addition, it should be noted that Pentacam should be used when using the A-P ratio of corneal curvature radius in the ISS method, and that the A-P ratio is not compatible with other instruments. We thank the authors again for their commentary on the evaluation methods of the multiple IOL frequency formulas used in this study.

Author Contributions: Writing—original draft, Y.I.; writing—review and editing, Y.I., K.S. and N.S. All authors have read and agreed to the published version of the manuscript.

Funding: This research received no external funding.

Institutional Review Board Statement: The study was conducted according to the guidelines of the Declaration of Helsinki and approved by the Institutional Review Board at the Kitasato University (protocol code B17-292) in 2018.

Informed Consent Statement: Informed consent was obtained from all subjects involved in the study.

Data Availability Statement: The data presented in this study are available on request from the corresponding author.

Conflicts of Interest: The authors declare no conflict of interest.

References

1. Cione, F.; De Bernardo, M.; Rosa, N. Comment on Iida et al. Development of a New Method for Calculating Intraocular Lens Power after Myopic Laser In Situ Keratomileusis by Combining the Anterior–Posterior Ratio of the Corneal Radius of the Curvature with the Double-K Method. *J. Clin. Med.* 2022, 11, 522. *J. Clin. Med.* **2022**, 11, 1996. [CrossRef] [PubMed]
2. Iida, Y.; Shimizu, K.; Shoji, N. Development of a New Method for Calculating Intraocular Lens Power after Myopic Laser In Situ Keratomileusis by Combining the Anterior–Posterior Ratio of the Corneal Radius of the Curvature with the Double-K Method. *J. Clin. Med.* **2022**, 11, 522. [CrossRef] [PubMed]
3. De Bernardo, M.; Iaccarino, S.; Cennamo, M.; Caliendo, L.; Rosa, N. Corneal Anterior Power Calculation for an IOL in Post-PRK Patients. *Optom. Vis. Sci.* **2015**, 92, 190–195. [CrossRef] [PubMed]
4. De Bernardo, M.; Borrelli, M.; Imparato, R.; Rosa, N. Calculation of the Real Corneal Refractive Power after Photorefractive Keratectomy Using Pentacam, When Only the Preoperative Refractive Error is Known. *J. Ophthalmol.* **2020**, 2020, 1916369. [CrossRef] [PubMed]
5. Rosa, N.; Cione, F.; Pepe, A.; Musto, S.; De Bernardo, M. An Advanced Lens Measurement Approach (ALMA) in post refractive surgery IOL power calculation with unknown preoperative parameters. *PLoS ONE* **2020**, 15, e0237990. [CrossRef] [PubMed]
6. Turnbull, A.M.J.; Crawford, G.J.; Barrett, G.D. Methods for Intraocular Lens Power Calculation in Cataract Surgery after Radial Keratotomy. *Ophthalmology* **2020**, 127, 45–51. [CrossRef] [PubMed]
7. Hoffer, K.J.; Savini, G. Update on Intraocular Lens Power Calculation Study Protocols: The Better Way to Design and Report Clinical Trials. *Ophthalmology* **2021**, 128, e115–e120. [CrossRef] [PubMed]
8. Saiki, M.; Negishi, K.; Kato, N.; Ogino, R.; Arai, H.; Toda, I.; Dogru, M.; Tsubota, K. Modified double-K method for intraocular lens power calculation after excimer laser corneal refractive surgery. *J. Cataract Refract. Surg.* **2013**, 39, 556–562. [CrossRef] [PubMed]
9. Abulafia, A.; Hill, W.E.; Koch, D.D.; Wang, L.; Barrett, G.D. Accuracy of the Barrett True-K Formula for Intraocular Lens Power Prediction after Laser In Situ Keratomileusis or Photorefractive Keratectomy for Myopia. *J. Cataract Refract. Surg.* **2016**, 42, 363–369. [CrossRef] [PubMed]

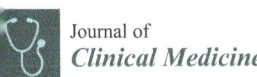

Review

Intraoperative Anterior Segment Optical Coherence Tomography in the Management of Cataract Surgery: State of the Art

Mario Damiano Toro [1,2], Serena Milan [3,*], Daniele Tognetto [3], Robert Rejdak [2], Ciro Costagliola [4], Sandrine Anne Zweifel [5], Chiara Posarelli [6], Michele Figus [6], Magdalena Rejdak [7], Teresio Avitabile [8], Adriano Carnevali [9,†] and Rosa Giglio [3,†]

1. Eye Clinic, Department of Public Health, University of Naples Federico II, 80131 Naples, Italy; toro.mario@email.it
2. Chair and Department of General and Pediatric Ophthalmology, Medical University of Lublin, 20079 Lublin, Poland; robert.rejdak@yahoo.com
3. Eye Clinic, Department of Medicine, Surgery and Health Sciences, University of Trieste, 34134 Trieste, Italy; tognetto@units.it (D.T.); giglio.rosam@gmail.com (R.G.)
4. Eye Clinic, Department of Neuroscience and Reproductive and Odontostomatological Sciences, University of Naples Federico II, 80131 Naples, Italy; ciro.costagliola1957@gmail.com
5. Department of Ophthalmology, University of Zurich, 8091 Zurich, Switzerland; sandrine.zweifel@usz.ch
6. Department of Surgical, Medical and Molecular Pathology and of Critical Care Medicine, University of Pisa, 56126 Pisa, Italy; chiara.posarelli@med.unipi.it (C.P.); michele.figus@unipi.it (M.F.)
7. Faculty of Medicine, Medical University of Warsaw, 02091 Warsaw, Poland; rejdakmagdalena@gmail.com
8. Department of Ophthalmology, University of Catania, 95124 Catania, Italy; t.avitabile@unict.it
9. Department of Ophthalmology, University Magna Graecia of Catanzaro, 88100 Catanzaro, Italy; adrianocarnevali@unicz.it
* Correspondence: serena.milan2@gmail.com
† These authors contributed equally to this work.

Abstract: Background: The introduction of non-invasive diagnostic tools in ophthalmology has significantly reshaped current clinical practice in different settings. Recently, different anterior segment (AS) intraoperative optical coherence tomography (i-OCT) systems have been employed for different interventional procedures including cataract surgery. Materials and Methods: A review on the use of AS i-OCT in the management of cataract surgery, following the Preferred Reporting Items for Systematic Reviews and Meta-Analyses guidelines (PRISMA). The level of evidence according to the Oxford Centre for Evidence-Based Medicine (OCEM) 2011 guidelines, and the quality of evidence according to the Grading of Recommendations Assessment, Development and Evaluation (GRADE) system were assessed for all included articles. Results: Out of 6302 articles initially extracted, 6302 abstracts were identified for screening and 32 of these met the inclusion/exclusion criteria for full-text review; 19 articles were excluded. Conclusions: The use of AS i-OCT in cataract surgery, even if only a few studies have a high level or grade of evidence, may represent a useful tool for novel surgeons approaching phacoemulsification but also for expert ones for teaching purposes and to plan and manage complicated cases.

Keywords: anterior segment OCT; intraoperative OCT; cataract surgery; surgical technique

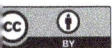

1. Introduction

Cataract surgery is one of the most cost-effective healthcare interventions. It affects both physical and psychological health [1,2] and it has undergone a significant modernization in the past fifty years [3]. Indeed, this procedure has been made effective and safe thanks to the introduction of minimally invasive techniques and the availability of innovative equipment.

Recently, intraoperative optical coherence tomography (i-OCT) systems have been integrated into ocular microscopes, providing useful feedback for the surgeons of both the anterior and posterior segments of the eye [4,5].

I-OCT is a non-invasive, real-time method with high resolution that can image the finest ocular structures even through mediums with significant opacity. However, to date the extent of the actual benefits of the application of i-OCT into common clinical practice is still debated [6].

This review aims at summarizing the current applications of anterior segment (AS) i-OCT in the management of cataract surgery while assessing the level and quality of the studies included in the review.

2. Materials and Methods

This systematic review was conducted and reported by the Preferred Reporting Items for Systematic Reviews and Meta-Analyses (PRISMA) guidelines [7]. The review protocol was not recorded in the study design, and no registration number is available for consultation. The methodology used for this comprehensive review consisted of a systematic search of all available articles exploring the use of AS i-OCT in patients undergoing cataract surgery. A literature search of all original articles published up to November 2021 was performed in parallel by two authors (MDT and MW) using the PubMed database.

The following terms were employed for "Cataract Extraction" (Mesh) OR "Refractive Errors" (Mesh) OR "Cataract" (Mesh) OR "Lens Implantation, Intraocular" (Mesh) OR "Anterior Eye Segment" (Mesh) AND "Tomography, Optical Coherence" (Mesh).

Furthermore, the reference lists of all identified articles were examined manually to identify any potential study not captured by the electronic searches. After the preparation of the list of all electronic data captured, two reviewers (MDT and MW) examined the titles and abstracts independently and identified relevant articles. Exclusion criteria were review studies, pilot studies, case series, case reports, photo essays, and studies written in languages other than English. Moreover, studies performed on animal eyes, cadaveric eyes and pediatric patients were excluded as well.

The same reviewers registered and selected the captured studies according to the inclusion and exclusion criteria by examining the full text of the articles. Any disagreement was assessed by consensus, and a third reviewer (MB) was consulted when necessary. No effort was made to contact the corresponding authors for further unpublished data. All selected articles were analyzed to assess the level of evidence according to the Oxford Centre for Evidence-Based Medicine (OCEM) 2011 guidelines [8], and the quality of evidence according to the Grading of Recommendations Assessment, Development and Evaluation (GRADE) system [9].

3. Results

The results of the search strategy are summarized in Figure 1. From 6302 articles extracted from the initial research, 6302 abstracts were identified for screening and 32 of these met the inclusion/exclusion criteria for full-text review. Nineteen articles were excluded (Figure 1).

Studies' characteristics, main results, level, and grade of the available evidence about the role of AS i-OCT in cataract surgery management are summarized in Table 1.

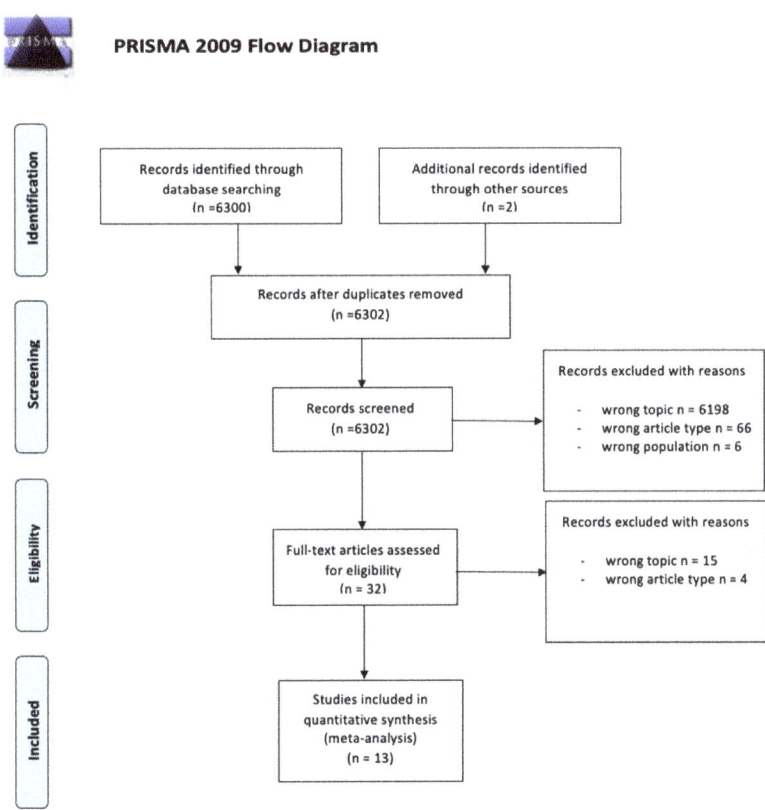

Figure 1. Flow diagram of the study according to Preferred Reporting Items for Systematic Reviews and Meta-Analyses (PRISMA) guidelines [7].

Table 1. Characteristics, quality, and level of evidence of the included studies and features of the anterior segment intraoperative optical coherence tomography (i-OCT) cited by these articles.

Author	Year	Study Design	Study Sample	Type of Surgery (n° of Eyes)	Type of Cataract (n°)	Intraoperative OCT (i-OCT) Specifications	Ocular Evaluation	Results	Grade [1]	Level [2]
Das S.	2016	Prospective study (P)	38 eyes (E)	Microincision cataract surgery (MICS) (28); femtosecond laser assisted cataract surgery (FLACS) (10)	Posterior polar cataracts (PPCs) (3); mature intumescent cataracts (2); nuclear cataracts (N) grade 2–3 (33).	RESCAN™ 700 (Carl Zeiss Meditec)	To describe the role of i-OCT in MICS and FLACS, focusing on wound assessment, hydroprocedures, nucleus management, intraocular lens (IOL) assessment	I-OCT could be useful for assessing wound morphology, deciding the adequate depth of trenching, and detecting intraocular lens (IOL) position.	Low	4
Tañá-Sanz P.	2021	P	102 E	FLACS	Not specified (NS)	Catalys (Johnson & Johnson Vision)	To compare different parameters obtained by i-OCT (before starting surgery) and preoperative OCT biometry.	Measurements provided by Catalys, IOLMaster 700 (Carl Zeiss Meditec) and Anterion (Heidelberg Engineering) are significantly different.	Low	4
Waring G.O. 4th	2020	Retrospective study (R)	293 E	FLACS (235); femtosecond laser-assisted refractive lens exchange (58)	NS	Catalys	To analyze the existing relationship among i-OCT-derived lens parameters, biometry, and age.	Commonly available biometric data couldn't predict i-OCT-derived lens parameters such as lens diameter and lens volume.	Moderate	4
Hirnschall N.	2013	P	70 E	MICS	NS	Visante (Carl Zeiss Meditec)	To analyze the potential role of i-OCT-derived parameters (acquired after crystalline lens removal) in prediction of postoperative IOL position	I-OCT measurement of anterior capsule position after capsular tension ring (CTR) insertion was a better predictor of the early postoperative IOL position compared with preoperative data.	Low	4
Kurosawa M.	2021	R	1070 E	FLACS	NS	Catalys	To study whether comparing preoperatively and intraoperatively acquired lens thickness (LT) could help in preventing surgical complications during nuclear laser irradiation in FLACS.	LT inspection could be useful to reduce inappropriate posterior capsule detection cases and consequently misdirected femtosecond laser spots.	Low	4
Palanker D.V.	2010	P	30 patients	MICS (30); FLACS (29)	N grade 1 to 4	Frequency-domain OCT (FD-OCT) model integrated on microscope	To develop a model of i-OCT-guided FLACS and to compare it with MICS, focusing on the capsulotomy step.	Capsulotomies performed by OCT-guided femtosecond lasers were characterized by sizes and shapes which were more similar to the intended ones than manual capsulorhexis.	Low	4
Titiyal J.S.	2018	P	129 E	MICS (77); FLACS (52)	NS	RESCAN™ 700	To evaluate the morphology of clear corneal incisions (CCIs) and their impact on Descemet membrane detachment (DMD).	A ragged morphology of CCIs was associated with a higher incidence of DMD; only i-OCT could detect an increase in its size or its development after stromal hydration.	Low	4

Table 1. Cont.

Author	Year	Study Design	Study Sample	Type of Surgery (n° of Eyes)	Type of Cataract (n°)	Intraoperative OCT (i-OCT) Specifications	Ocular Evaluation	Results	Grade[1]	Level[2]
Song V.K.	2019	R	35 (E)	FLACS	NS	Catalys	To study the anatomical overlap between the pupil center (PC), the limbal center (LC) and the lens center, in order to guide capsulotomy.	The PC was nearer to the lens center than the LC.	Very low	4
Mastropasqua L.	2014	P	90 E	Lensx (Alcon Laboratories) FLACS (30); Lensar (Lensar) FLACS (30); MICS (30).	NS	Lensx; Lensar	To compare capsulotomies obtained with FLACS with manual capsulorhexis.	FLACS capsulotomies were greater than manual ones, determining a more precise IOL centration.	Moderate	3
Titiyal J.S.	2020	P	50 E	MICS	White cataracts	RESCAN™ 700	To analyze white cataract morphology and intraoperative dynamics, focusing on capsulorhexis.	I-OCT permitted the identification of four types of white cataracts, based on their anatomical characteristics and surgical behavior during capsulorhexis, helping the surgeon dealing with rhexis' extension-related complications.	Low	4
Titiyal J.S.	2020	P; R	112 E	MICS	PPCs	RESCAN™ 700	To evaluate the morphology of PPCs, intraoperative dynamics of the posterior capsule and the occurrence of posterior capsular dehiscence.	I-OCT could help in detecting those PPCs which could undergo safe hydrodissection.	Low	4
Anisimova N.S.	2020	P	28 videos	MICS (13); FLACS (15)	N	RESCAN™ 700	To identify the presence of incomplete vitreolenticular adhesion, immediately after IOL implantation.	I-OCT permitted the identification of undesired particles into Berger's space with a higher sensitivity than post-operative OCT.	Very low	4
Juergens L.	2021	P	4 E	Standard phacoemulsification combined with iris diaphragm implantation	NS	EnFocus Ultra-Deep OCT (Leica Microsystems)	To assess when the use of i-OCT could be relevant for intra-operative procedures.	I-OCT was crucial for the implantation of a two-part brown iris diaphragm, because of the poor contrast between the anterior lens capsule margin and the brown implant.	Very low	5

[1] Quality of evidence according to the Grading of Recommendations Assessment, Development and Evaluation (GRADE) system [9]. [2] Level of evidence according to the Oxford Centre for Evidence-Based Medicine (OCEM) 2011 guidelines [8].

No data synthesis was possible for the heterogeneity of available data and the design of the available studies. Thus, the current review reports a qualitative analysis, detailed issue-by-issue below narratively.

The i-OCT visualization of ocular changes occurring during cataract surgery (both standard and femtosecond-laser-assisted using LenSx Laser System -Alcon Laboratories was described by Das et al. [10]. The i-OCT employed was the RESCAN™ 700 (Carl Zeiss Meditec), which is a 3 dimensional (3D) spectral-domain OCT (SD-OCT) characterized by a wavelength of 840 nm, an axial resolution of 5.5 µm, and an A-scan depth of 2000 µm. Continuous video monitoring permitted assessment of wound morphology (length, breadth number of planes, epithelium disruption, amount of wound gape, endothelial alignment Descemet membrane detachment-DMD) and wound closure adequacy (corneal stroma whitening and thickening induced by hydration of the side port and the main incision was qualitatively estimated), to visualize capsulorhexis, to clearly monitor hydrodissection and hydrodelineation procedures. Interestingly in two out of three posterior polar cataracts (PCCs), the opacity could be clearly distinguished from the posterior capsule and a safe hydrodissection was performed. Moreover, they applied i-OCT to image the distention of the capsular bag during intumescent cataract surgery, to decide the exact depth of trenching and to assess the amount of wound distortion during intraocular lens (IOL) implantation to check the final IOL position.

Tañá-Sanz et al. studied four AS parameters obtained intraoperatively with the i-OCT integrated into the Catalys (Johnson & Johnson Vision) femtosecond laser platform which is an AS SD-OCT characterized by a central wavelength of 820–930 nm and an axial resolution of <30 µm [11]. The parameters included in the analysis were anterior chamber depth (ACD), central corneal thickness (CCT), lens thickness (LT), and white-to-white (WTW). They compared these parameters with those acquired preoperatively with two swept-source OCT (SS-OCT) biometers (IOLMaster 700-Carl Zeiss Meditec- and Anterion Heidelberg Engineering). Statistically significant differences were shown for all parameters with the Catalys being associated with the greatest values of ACD (mean difference with Anterion: +0.183 ± 0.056 mm; mean difference with IOL Master 700: +0.250 ± 0.054 mm), CCT (mean difference with Anterion: +32.110 ± 9.347 µm; mean difference with IOL Master 700: +24.473 ± 10.897 µm) and LT (mean difference with Anterion: +0.026 ± 0.024 mm mean difference with IOL Master 700: +0.088 ± 0.029 mm) and the shortest WTW (mean difference with Anterion: −0.236 ± 0.604 mm; mean difference with IOL Master 700 −0.385 ± 0.575 mm).

Waring et al. used Catalys' i-OCT to study possible correlations among ACD, LT, lens diameter (LD, the distance from the intersections of the anterior to posterior lens surfaces) and lens volume (LV, the volume of the lens calculated from the measured anterior and posterior lenticular surface curvatures that were extended to intersect in the lenticular periphery) [12]. While ACD and LT could be easily detected, LD and LV could be acquired only by i-OCT and were related to lens aging. It was found that LV had a strong positive correlation with both LT and LD; all three lens anatomy parameters demonstrated a positive correlation with age (moderate for LT and LV, weak for LD). ACD showed a moderate inverse correlation with LT, a weak positive correlation with LD, and a weak inverse correlation with LV. Biometric data obtained with IOL Master 500 (Carl Zeiss Meditec) were also included. AL had a weak correlation with LD, a weak inverse correlation with LT, and no correlation with LV. The authors provided regression equations to predict LD and LV from conventionally available parameters (AL, ACD, LT, age, average WTW, and average keratometry).

Hirnschall et al. studied if intraoperative lens capsule position after crystalline lens removal could represent a useful parameter to predict IOL position [13]. A capsular tension ring (CTR) was introduced in all patients to cause a taut and straight planar posterior capsule. They used a prototype of an AS time-domain OCT (Visante-Carl Zeiss Meditec-characterized by a wavelength of 1310 nm and an axial resolution of 18 um) combined with an operating microscope. During surgery, four screenshots were taken: at the beginning of surgery, after irrigation/aspiration (I/A) of cortical material and Ophthalmic Viscosurgical Device (OVD) removal, after implantation of a CTR, and at the end of surgery. Intraoperative parameters were combined with ACD values acquired preoperatively, 1 hour after surgery, and three months postoperatively with PCI meter (Carl Zeiss Meditec), IOLMaster 500, and ACMaster (Carl Zeiss Meditec). Regarding immediate postoperative ACD, the position of the anterior capsule post-CTR insertion (CTRa) was associated with the highest variable importance projection (VIP), followed by the position of the anterior lens capsule after lens removal without a CTR, whereas the posterior lens capsule was a poor predictor. Regarding 1 hour after surgery ACD, it was found that AL and CTRa were excellent predictors, preoperative ACD was good, while LT was poor. AL, CTRa, and preoperatively measured ACD turned out to be excellent predictors of three-month after surgery ACD, while LT was a poor predictor.

In their study, Kurosawa et al. reported a case of posterior capsule dehiscence induced by misdirected laser irradiation, caused by the detection of a high OCT intensity area in the anterior vitreous (misinterpreted as the posterior capsule) [14]. They consequently proposed a method to avoid this complication, called LT inspection: it stands for comparing pre-operative LT (detected with IOL Master 700 and CASIA2, TOMEY) with intraoperative LT (detected with Catalys' i-OCT) before laser irradiation and, eventually, to manually correct intraoperative data based on this comparison. A total of 546 patients underwent LT inspection: in one case, an inappropriate posterior capsule line was shown, and LT inspection avoided its break. Additionally, 474 patients were retrospectively analyzed, and it was found that four patients (including the previously mentioned case of posterior capsule dehiscence) had an inappropriate posterior capsule detection. However, the "posterior capsular safety margin" (which is a laser setting) of 500 μm avoided the complication in three out of four patients.

Palanker et al. developed a system combining a frequency-domain OCT (FD-OCT, characterized by an axial resolution of 11 mm) with a femtosecond laser system [15]. They made a comparison of laser capsulotomies and manual capsulorhexis in terms of size (measured along the x and y axes, repeated after rotation by 45°) and shape (the circularity was measured as a ratio of the sample area to the area of a disk with a diameter corresponding to the greatest linear dimension of the sample—this ratio is equal to 1 in an ideal circle). Measurements were obtained during surgery right after the capsular disk removal (with a Seibel Rhexis ruler), on the extracted capsule (after removal, they were put between glass slides, stained with 0.5% trypan blue, and then digital light microscopy was performed), and based on the digital images obtained during slit lamp exam one week and one month after surgery. Deviation from the intended size was -282 ± 305 μm in manual capsulorhexis and 27 ± 25 μm in laser capsulotomy. Concerning circularity, they calculated a 0.77 ± 0.15 ratio for manual capsulorhexis, and a 0.95 ± 0.04 ratio for the laser ones.

Titiyal et al. applied the i-OCT integrated on RESCAN™ 700 to study the correlation between morphological characteristics of clear corneal incisions (CCIs) and the incidence of intraoperative DMD, comparing conventional phacoemulsification to femtosecond laser-assisted cataract surgery (FLACS) [16]. Firstly, CCIs internal slit openings were classified by a single surgeon under the operating microscope, at the beginning of surgery before the occurrence of DMD, as ragged slit (RS, irregular wavy appearance) or smooth slit (SS, SS-like uniform appearance). RS morphology was observed in 31.2% of cases of the conventional surgery group and in 13.5% of cases of the FLACS group. Then, incision sites were assessed after incision creation, after phacoemulsification, after irrigation-aspiration, after IOL insertion, and after stromal hydration: DMD was described when Descemet membrane separation from the underlying stroma was visible on i-OCT or both i-OCT and the operating microscope. Forty-three out of 129 cases experienced localized incision-site DMD; incidence was significantly higher in cases with RS morphology (87.1%) than SS morphology (16.3%). All DMDs detected by i-OCT were also detectable under the operating microscope before stromal hydration; however, only i-OCT could detect an increase in its size or its onset after stromal hydration (which represented the phase in which the higher rate of DMD occurred-83.7% cases). Incision sites were also checked one day and thirty days after surgery using slit-lamp biomicroscopy and AS-OCT (RTVue-100; Optovue): at day 30, incision-site DMD wasn't detectable in any case.

Song et al. analyzed the location of the pupil center (PC), the limbal center (LC), and the lens center (which can be extrapolated from the location of anterior and posterior lens capsule lines) with Catalys's i-OCT in patients undergoing FLACS [17]. Angle K (consequently, the location of the visual axis-VA) was acquired preoperatively with OPD scan III (Nidek). Lens center-LC distance was 0.205 ± 0.104 mm, lens center-VA distance was 0.296 ± 0.198 mm, while lens center-PC distance was 0.147 ± 0.103 mm (the smallest one); the LC was located significantly inferiorly and temporally compared to the PC. In regards to distances from the VA, the PC had a distance of 0.283 ± 0.161 mm, the LC of 0.362 ± 0.153 mm, and the lens center of 0.296 ± 0.198 mm.

In their study, Mastropasqua et al. studied capsulorhexis features after FLACS and manual cataract surgery [18]. Enrolled patients were randomly divided into three groups: patients of the first group underwent FLACS with Lensx platform (high-definition OCT visualization system), and for the second group Lenstar (Lenstar) FLACS was applied (which is guided by an integrated 3D confocal structured imaging system), while the standard manual technique was used for the last group. Regarding capsulotomy circularity, in the first seven days after surgery it was statistically significantly better in laser groups, but no statistically significant differences were observed at 30 days and 180 days. At all time points, the manual capsulorhexis area was significantly smaller than the laser one. Laser capsulotomies were also associated with a statistically significantly lower deviation from the intended size. In regards to the distance between the pupil centroid and IOL centroid, it was statistically significantly lower in laser groups than in the manual group; the distance between the pupil centroid and capsulotomy was also statistically significantly lower in laser groups than in the manual group.

Titiyal et al. analyzed morphological features and intraoperative behavior of white cataracts with RESCAN™ 700 i-OCT [19]. Regarding surgical steps, capsulorhexis was done under a cohesive OVD (starting with a 26-gauge bent needle cystotome and ending using a micro forceps or needle cystotome based on the intraoperative characteristics). Bimanual I/A of cortical material was needed if an impending risk of capsulorhexis escape was detected. Difficulties in capsulorhexis were subjectively assessed by the operating surgeon based on the surgeon's control over the size and circularity of the rhexis while performing the anterior capsular flap tear. After gentle hydrodissection, nuclear emulsification and eventually I/A were performed, ending with IOL implantation. Four kinds of cataracts were described: type I (characterized by regularly organized cortical fibers), type II (with a more convex anterior capsule and multiple intralenticular clefts), type III (in which the convexity of the anterior capsule and the clefts were combined with areas of homogeneous ground glass appearance), and type IV (in which the anterior lens cortex had a homogeneous ground-glass appearance). Type I underwent uncomplicated capsulorhexis; in type II cataracts, i-OCT showed a cortical bulge in the anterior chamber during initial nick creation, standing for raised intralenticular pressure with a high risk of rhexis extension and leading the surgeon to perform a bimanual I/A till its lowering; regarding type III and type IV, the lowering of intralenticular pressure was observed at the beginning of the rhexis, outlining an increased risk of extension.

Titiyal et al. also analyzed morphological features of PPCs during standard phacoemulsification by using RESCAN™ 700 i-OCT [20]. At the beginning of surgery, i-OCT was used to assess the morphology of PPC (observed as a hyperreflective region in the posterior pole area), the relation of the opacity to the posterior capsule (which appears as a continuous hyperechoic concave line limiting the posterior aspect of the nucleus) and integrity and continuity of the posterior capsule. After hydrodelineation, the relation between posterior capsule and epinuclear cushion was valued to notice any posterior capsule-epinucleus fluid interface causing accidental hydrodissection. Three types of PPCs were consequently described: type I was characterized by an intact posterior capsule visualized along the entirety of the posterior polar opacity, with rly d from the capsule; in type II, the dense central region of PPC was apparently adherent to the posterior capsule, which could be detected only in the periphery; in type III the posterior capsule status couldn't be analyzed at all. The preoperative AS-OCT features correlated with the i-OCT features. Type I underwent gentle hydrodissection in addition to hydrodelineation and intraoperative posterior capsule break never occurred; type II and III underwent just hydrodelineation. Accidental hydrodissection occurred in 1 PPC type II during hydrodelineation; however, the posterior capsule remained intact till the end of surgery. Moreover, the incidence of capsule dehiscence in these i-OCT-guided surgeries (7.5%) was also retrospectively compared to not i-OCT-guided surgeries (11.1%) and statistically significant differences were noted.

Anisimova et al. studied the Berger space during and after 15 FLACS and 13 standard phacoemulsifications [6]. Videos were recorded immediately after IOL implantation (through the application of i-OCT integrated on RESCAN ™) and in the early postoperative period (with the RTVue XR 100, Optovue). Berger space was detected in 75% of cases intraoperatively and in 82% of cases postoperatively; in 32% of cases postoperatively, it was occupied by hyperreflective spots and particles, while i-OCT turned out to be more sensitive (57% of cases).

Juergens et al. described the potential benefits of i-OCT during 29 surgical procedures, among which four were cataract surgeries [21]. They employed EnFocus Ultra-Deep OCT (Leica Microsystems) integrated into the microscope, characterized by a maximum penetration depth of 11 mm, a maximum axial resolution of 9 µm, and a maximum lateral resolution of 15–31 µm. The authors described the case of a patient requiring additional implantation of a two-part, brown iris diaphragm because of post-neuro-borreliosis maximum pupillary rigidity, stating that only i-OCT imaging could assess iris diaphragm position in the capsule sac because of the poor contrast between the anterior lens capsule margin and the brown implant.

4. Discussion

The introduction of i-OCT-integrated surgical microscopes might represent a further step toward a safer and more efficient surgery. To date, different i-OCT systems can be integrated into an ocular microscope, providing useful feedback for the surgeons both the anterior and posterior segment surgeons [22,23].

When dealing with AS procedures, this technology provides direct visualization of anatomic structures before, during, and after surgical maneuvers, allows for an analysis of surgical planes, guides surgical steps, and helps to detect intraoperative complications, eventually impacting surgical decision-making [5,24,25].

In their study, Tañá-Sanz et al. demonstrated that some AS parameters (ACD, CCT, LT, and WTW) obtained with the AS-SD-OCT integrated into the Catalys femtosecond laser platform differed from those derived from SS-OCT biometers (IOLMaster 700 and Anterion biometer). According to the authors, these differences could be related to patients' position and the mydriasis required for the surgery [11].

In addition to these parameters, which can be easily acquired by traditional biometry, a greater understanding of lens anatomy (including the dimensions of the aged crystalline lens and its capsule) could be useful for surgeons and the development of new IOL formulas and technologies. However, most studies have been conducted in research settings, applying customized devices and not commonly available instruments (such as Magnetic Resonance Imaging), consequently, results couldn't be easily applied to clinical practice. Moreover, the ability of more commonly available biometric data to predict LD and LV is quite limited. The introduction of i-OCT integrated on femtosecond laser platforms has facilitated the study of lens anatomy in larger data sets making new lens parameters, consequently, available [26]. In their work, Waring et al. showed that i-OCT could detect LV, LD, and LT and they provided regression equations to predict LD and LV from conventionally available parameters. The authors stated this additional info could help in effective lens position (ELP) estimate/ion (consequently improving IOL power calculation and enhancing refractive predictability) and, in new IOL technologies development, such as capsule refilling [12].

Indeed, the prediction of the IOL position after surgery still represents one of the main issues when dealing with IOL power calculation [27,28].

Hirnshall et al. analyzed if intraoperative lens measurements, instead of preoperative ACD measurements, could improve ELP evaluation. It was found that the position of the anterior capsule after the insertion of a CTR represented an excellent predictor of ACD before surgery. However, it must be stated that to acquire these values, the use of a CTR was required (which is not an ordinary step in uncomplicated surgery) and that preoperative AL and ACD were also associated with high VIP for the prediction of ACD measured three months after surgery [13].

In cataract surgery, i-OCT might represent a valid device both for standard phacoemulsification procedures and for FLACS. Its main applications include the visualization of corneal incisions and the stromal hydration, the assessment of hydro-dissection, perception of the trenching depth, and identification of lens positioning [10,29]. Thus, the use of i-OCT might allow a safer surgical procedure, decreasing the rate of postoperative wound leak and hypotony and preventing any iatrogenic capsular rupture during hydro-dissection and phacoemulsification [22,24].

Titiyal et al. compared the morphology of CCIs in conventional phacoemulsification and FLACS using i-OCT; they noticed that a ragged slit morphology was a significant predictive factor for incision site DMD and it occurred more frequently during conventional surgery. Interestingly, the authors stated that all DMDs detected by i-OCT were also detectable under the operating microscope before stromal hydration; however, an increase in the extent of DMD or the occurrence of DMD after stromal hydration (which represented the phase in which the higher rate of DMD occurred—83.7% cases) were only detected by i-OCT. At any rate, all DMDs solved spontaneously in one month without requiring additional surgery [16]. The ability to detect an early subclinical DMD, an epithelial disruption, or a microtear in the inner or outer lip of the wound intraoperatively could be of great value for the surgeon not only to modify the subsequent steps of surgery but also to manage the early post-operative period [10].

The location of the Continuous curvilinear capsulorhexis (CCC) is critical for visual outcomes [30,31]. In conventional cataract surgery, the procedure is guided by the position of the PC and the LC, which are easily detected using a microscope; in FLACS, they can automatically be detected, together with an additional parameter called lens center. This represents very interesting data since the IOL center position will be similar to the center of the crystalline lens. A precisely sized and centered capsulotomy, enabled by this method might improve predictability and control of the IOL placement reducing IOL tilting and decentration. Song et al. analyzed the relative location of and distance between the PC, the LC, and the lens center in patients who underwent FLACS. It was found that the PC was closer to the lens center than the LC whose X and Y coordinate position was significantly inferior and temporal compared to the PC [17,32].

Palanker et al. compared the size and the shape of laser capsulotomy to manual ones using a system combining FD-OCT with a femtosecond pattern scanning laser. They demonstrated that the former was characterized by size more similar to the intended one than the latter; moreover, they were more circular than manual ones [15].

Mastropasqua et al. analyzed the characteristics of capsulotomies obtained during two types of i-OCT guided FLACS platforms (Lensx and Lensar) and during a standard manual technique. Laser-made capsulotomies demonstrated significantly better circularity than the manual CCCs at seven days, their sizes were much more similar to the intended ones, and they showed greater IOLs centration than the manual group at all time points [18].

As for biometry images, optical opacity could also affect the quality of i-OCT images leading to misleading analysis. During FLACS, precise detection of radiation sites is critical to correct the direction of spots and to avoid complications. Kurosawa et al. demonstrated that LT inspection could guide the surgeon in adjusting laser settings and avoiding posterior capsule breaks [14].

Moreover, real-time visualization of the trenching depth during phacoemulsification could be very useful for surgeons in training to decide the exact location to crack the nucleus during divide and conquer techniques [10].

Many authors have underlined the importance of i-OCT in complicated cases [33]. When dealing with white cataracts, the direct visualization of lens anatomical features through i-OCT could help anticipate the intraoperative dynamics of spontaneous milky fluid release, thus letting the surgeon be ready to deal with possible complications, especially during capsulorhexis [19].

For traumatic cataracts or PPCs, i-OCT could identify a capsular defect preventing further complications for the surgeon [20,29,34]. PPCs still represent a surgical challenge [35], due to the high incidence of posterior capsular break. To prevent it, hydrodissection is commonly avoided, consequently requiring greater manipulations during cortical clean-up and longer surgical time. In their study, Titiyal et al. evaluated morphological characteristics and intraoperative dynamics of PPCs with i-OCT, demonstrating that in the case of an intact posterior capsule homogenously spaced from the posterior polar opacity (called "type I PPC") gentle hydrodissection could be safely performed. At any rate, the authors declared the preoperative AS-OCT features correlated with the intraoperative ones. Moreover, according to the authors, i-OCT use didn't reduce the incidence of posterior capsule dehiscence compared to not i-OCT-guided surgeries [20].

I-OCT could also be helpful in patients with ectopia lentis, preventing further corneal endothelium damage during lens removal [36,37].

Juergens et al. reported i-OCT to be crucial for the implantation of a two-part brown iris diaphragm, because of the poor contrast between the anterior lens capsule margin and the brown implant [21].

Interestingly, i-OCT could detect the presence of direct intraoperative communication between Berger space and anterior chamber, which might lead to excessive fluid flow through this segment causing anterior displacement of the posterior capsule thus increasing the risk for a posterior capsular break and iris prolapse. Anisimova et al. showed that i-OCT could identify the presence of lens micro fragments and cellular material within the Berger space for the discontinuity of the zonules and Wieger ligament, with a higher sensitivity than postoperative OCT. Furthermore, they hypothesized that Wieger ligament detachment was associated with increased zonular permeability. This observation could be useful to clarify the mechanism of acute aqueous misdirection syndrome also known as acute rock-hard eye syndrome (AIRES) [6].

Although i-OCT might represent a helpful and not invasive tool, its application in clinical practice presents several limitations for cataract surgery. Firstly, intraoperative measurements are still time-consuming. Secondly, OCT-friendly instruments to reduce shadowing and integrated calipers are still lacking [10,13]. Moreover, total cataracts or extremely dense nuclear sclerosis reduce the ability of i-OCT to visualize the posterior capsule [19,20]. Finally, the analysis of the intraoperative images is not automatic, and it is still influenced too much by the insights of the observer.

5. Conclusions

In summary, the use of i-OCT in cataract surgery may represent a useful tool for novel surgeons approaching phacoemulsification, but also for expert ones for teaching purposes and to plan and manage complicated cases. I-OCT could also be employed to avoid refractive errors or intraoperative complications in patients with white cataracts or PPCs and to identify micro fragments in the Berger space. However, only a few studies have shown a sufficient grade or level of evidence and some limitations have been pointed out. Prospective studies would be ideal to pursue the question of the advantages of the use of i-OCT in cataract surgery and the factors or conditions that may indicate its use.

Author Contributions: Conceptualization, M.D.T., R.G. and A.C.; methodology, M.D.T., R.G. and A.C.; software, validation, formal analysis, investigation, resources, data curation, all authors; writing—original draft preparation, M.D.T., R.G., A.C. and S.M.; writing—review and editing, all authors; visualization, all authors; supervision, all authors; project administration, M.D.T.; funding acquisition, M.D.T. and R.R. All authors have read and agreed to the published version of the manuscript.

Funding: This research received no external funding.

Institutional Review Board Statement: Not applicable.

Informed Consent Statement: Not applicable.

Data Availability Statement: Data are available on reasonable request by the corresponding author.

Acknowledgments: The work-study has been supported by the "Foundation to support the development of Ophthalmology", Lublin, Poland. The Foundation had no role in the interpretation of data or in the decision to publish the results.

Conflicts of Interest: The authors declare no conflict of interest.

References

1. Wang, W.; Yan, W.; Fotis, K.; Prasad, N.M.; Lansingh, V.C.; Taylor, H.R.; Finger, R.P.; Facciolo, D.; He, M. Cataract Surgical Rate and Socioeconomics: A Global Study. *Investig. Ophthalmol. Vis. Sci.* **2016**, *57*, 5872–5881. [CrossRef] [PubMed]
2. Tognetto, D.; Brézin, A.P.; Cummings, A.B.; Malyugin, B.E.; Kemer, O.E.; Prieto, I.; Rejdak, R.; Teus, M.A.; Törnblom, R.; Toro, M.D.; et al. Rethinking Elective Cataract Surgery Diagnostics, Assessments, and Tools after the COVID-19 Pandemic Experience and Beyond: Insights from the EUROCOVCAT Group. *Diagnostics* **2020**, *10*, 1035. [CrossRef] [PubMed]
3. Leon, P.; Umari, I.; Mangogna, A.; Zanei, A.; Tognetto, D. An evaluation of intraoperative and postoperative outcomes of torsional mode versus longitudinal ultrasound mode phacoemulsification: A Meta-analysis. *Int. J. Ophthalmol.* **2016**, *9*, 890–897. [CrossRef] [PubMed]
4. Chisari, C.G.; Toro, M.D.; Cimino, V.; Rejdak, R.; Luca, M.; Rapisarda, L.; Avitabile, T.; Posarelli, C.; Rejdak, K.; Reibaldi, M.; et al. Retinal Nerve Fiber Layer Thickness and Higher Relapse Frequency May Predict Poor Recovery after Optic Neuritis in MS Patients. *J. Clin. Med.* **2019**, *8*, 2022. [CrossRef] [PubMed]
5. Posarelli, C.; Sartini, F.; Casini, G.; Passani, A.; Toro, M.D.; Vella, G.; Figus, M. What Is the Impact of Intraoperative Microscope-Integrated OCT in Ophthalmic Surgery? Relevant Applications and Outcomes. A Systematic Review. *J. Clin. Med.* **2020**, *9*, 1682. [CrossRef]
6. Anisimova, N.; Arbisser, L.B.; Shilova, N.F.; A Melnik, M.; Belodedova, A.V.; Knyazer, B.; E Malyugin, B. Anterior vitreous detachment: Risk factor for intraoperative complications during phacoemulsification. *J. Cataract Refract. Surg.* **2020**, *46*, 55–62. [PubMed]
7. Moher, D.; Liberati, A.; Tetzlaff, J.; Altman, D.G.; PRISMA Group. Preferred reporting items for systematic reviews and meta-analyses: The PRISMA statement. *PLoS Med.* **2009**, *6*, e1000097. [CrossRef]
8. Howick, J.; Glasziou, P.; Aronson, J.K. Evidence-based mechanistic reasoning. *J. R. Soc. Med.* **2010**, *103*, 433–441. [CrossRef]
9. Guyatt, G.; Oxman, A.D.; Akl, E.A.; Kunz, R.; Vist, G.; Brozek, J.; Norris, S.; Falck-Ytter, Y.; Glasziou, P.; DeBeer, H.; et al. GRADE guidelines: 1. Introduction—GRADE evidence profiles and summary of findings tables. *J. Clin. Epidemiol.* **2011**, *64*, 383–394. [CrossRef]
10. Das, S.; Kummelil, M.K.; Kharbanda, V.; Arora, V.; Nagappa, S.; Shetty, R.; Shetty, B.K. Microscope Integrated Intraoperative Spectral Domain Optical Coherence Tomography for Cataract Surgery: Uses and Applications. *Curr. Eye Res.* **2015**, *41*, 643–652. [CrossRef]
11. Tañá-Sanz, P.; Ruiz-Santos, M.; Rodríguez-Carrillo, M.D.; Aguilar-Córcoles, S.; Montés-Micó, R.; Tañá-Rivero, P. Agreement between intraoperative anterior segment spectral-domain OCT and 2 swept-source OCT biometers. *Expert Rev. Med. Devices* **2021**, *18*, 387–393. [CrossRef] [PubMed]
12. Waring, G.O.; Chang, D.H.; Rocha, K.M.; Gouvea, L.; Penatti, R. Correlation of Intraoperative Optical Coherence Tomography of Crystalline Lens Diameter, Thickness, and Volume with Biometry and Age. *Am. J. Ophthalmol.* **2020**, *225*, 147–156. [CrossRef] [PubMed]
13. Hirnschall, N.; Amir-Asgari, S.; Maedel, S.; Findl, O. Predicting the Postoperative Intraocular Lens Position Using Continuous Intraoperative Optical Coherence Tomography Measurements. *Investig. Opthalmol. Vis. Sci.* **2013**, *54*, 5196–5203. [CrossRef] [PubMed]
14. Kurosawa, M.; Horiguchi, H.; Shiba, T.; Nakano, T. Inspection of the lens thickness with preoperative biometric measurements prevents an erroneous interpretation of posterior capsule during FLACS. *Sci. Rep.* **2021**, *11*, 1–7. [CrossRef]
15. Palanker, D.V.; Blumenkranz, M.S.; Andersen, D.; Wiltberger, M.; Marcellino, G.; Gooding, P.; Angeley, D.; Schuele, G.; Woodley, B.; Simoneau, M.; et al. Femtosecond Laser–Assisted Cataract Surgery with Integrated Optical Coherence Tomography. *Sci. Transl. Med.* **2010**, *2*, 58ra85. [CrossRef]

6. Titiyal, J.S.; Kaur, M.; Ramesh, P.; Shah, P.; Falera, R.; Bageshwar, L.M.S.; Kinkar, A.; Sharma, N. Impact of Clear Corneal Incision Morphology on Incision-Site Descemet Membrane Detachment in Conventional and Femtosecond Laser-Assisted Phacoemulsification. *Curr. Eye Res.* **2017**, *43*, 293–299. [CrossRef]
7. Song, W.K.; Lee, J.A.; Kim, J.Y.; Kim, M.J.; Tchah, H. Analysis of Positional Relationships of Various Centers in Cataract Surgery. *Korean J. Ophthalmol.* **2019**, *33*, 70–81. [CrossRef]
8. Mastropasqua, L.; Toto, L.; Mattei, P.A.; Vecchiarino, L.; Mastropasqua, A.; Navarra, R.; Di Nicola, M.; Nubile, M. Optical coherence tomography and 3-dimensional confocal structured imaging system–guided femtosecond laser capsulotomy versus manual continuous curvilinear capsulorhexis. *J. Cataract Refract. Surg.* **2014**, *40*, 2035–2043. [CrossRef]
9. Titiyal, J.S.; Kaur, M.; Shaikh, F.; Goel, S.; Bageshwar, L.M.S. Real-time intraoperative dynamics of white cataract—intraoperative optical coherence tomography–guided classification and management. *J. Cataract Refract. Surg.* **2020**, *46*, 598–605. [CrossRef]
10. Titiyal, J.S.; Kaur, M.; Shaikh, F.; Rani, D.; Bageshwar, L.M. Elucidating intraoperative dynamics and safety in posterior polar cataract with intraoperative OCT-guided phacoemulsification. *J. Cataract Refract. Surg.* **2020**, *46*, 1266–1272. [CrossRef]
11. Juergens, L.; Michiels, S.; Borrelli, M.; Spaniol, K.; Guthoff, R.; Schrader, S.; Frings, A.; Geerling, G. Intraoperative OCT—Real-World User Evaluation in Routine Surgery. *Klin. Mon. Augenheilkd.* **2021**, *238*, 693–699. [CrossRef] [PubMed]
12. Ehlers, J.P. Intraoperative optical coherence tomography: Past, present, and future. *Eye* **2015**, *30*, 193–201. [CrossRef] [PubMed]
13. Ehlers, J.P.; Dupps, W.; Kaiser, P.; Goshe, J.; Singh, R.P.; Petkovsek, D.; Srivastava, S.K. The Prospective Intraoperative and Perioperative Ophthalmic ImagiNg with Optical CoherEncE TomogRaphy (PIONEER) Study: 2-Year Results. *Am. J. Ophthalmol.* **2014**, *158*, 999–1007.e1. [CrossRef]
14. Lu, C.D.; Waheed, N.K.; Witkin, A.; Baumal, C.R.; Liu, J.J.; Potsaid, B.; Joseph, A.; Jayaraman, V.; Cable, A.; Chan, K.; et al. Microscope-Integrated Intraoperative Ultrahigh-Speed Swept-Source Optical Coherence Tomography for Widefield Retinal and Anterior Segment Imaging. *Ophthalmic Surg. Lasers Imaging Retin.* **2018**, *49*, 94–102. [CrossRef] [PubMed]
15. Dick, H.B.; Schultz, T. Primary Posterior Laser-Assisted Capsulotomy. *J. Refract. Surg.* **2014**, *30*, 128–134. [CrossRef] [PubMed]
16. Haddad, J.S.; Rocha, K.M.; Yeh, K.; Iv, G.O.W. Lens anatomy parameters with intraoperative spectral-domain optical coherence tomography in cataractous eyes. *Clin. Ophthalmol.* **2019**, *13*, 253–260. [CrossRef] [PubMed]
17. Hirnschall, N.; Norrby, S.; Weber, M.; Maedel, S.; Amir-Asgari, S.; Findl, O. Using continuous intraoperative optical coherence tomography measurements of the aphakic eye for intraocular lens power calculation. *Br. J. Ophthalmol.* **2014**, *99*, 7–10. [CrossRef]
18. Lytvynchuk, L.M.; Glittenberg, C.G.; Falkner-Radler, C.I.; Neumaier-Ammerer, B.; Smretschnig, E.; Hagen, S.; Ansari-Shahrezaei, S.; Binder, S. Evaluation of intraocular lens position during phacoemulsification using intraoperative spectral-domain optical coherence tomography. *J. Cataract Refract. Surg.* **2016**, *42*, 694–702. [CrossRef]
19. Yadav, S.; Mukhija, R.; Pujari, A.; Tandon, R. Intraoperative optical coherence tomography-guided assessment of hydro-dissection procedure during cataract surgery. *Indian J. Ophthalmol.* **2020**, *68*, 1647–1648. [CrossRef]
20. Bala, C.; Chan, T.; Meades, K. Factors affecting corneal incision position during femtosecond laser–assisted cataract surgery. *J. Cataract Refract. Surg.* **2017**, *43*, 1541–1548. [CrossRef]
21. Hirasawa, H.; Murata, H.; Mayama, C.; Araie, M.; Asaoka, R. Evaluation of various machine learning methods to predict vision-related quality of life from visual field data and visual acuity in patients with glaucoma. *Br. J. Ophthalmol.* **2014**, *98*, 1230–1235. [CrossRef] [PubMed]
22. Schultz, T.; Tsiampalis, N.; Dick, H.B. Laser-Assisted Capsulotomy Centration: A Prospective Trial Comparing Pupil Versus OCT-Based Scanned Capsule Centration. *J. Refract. Surg.* **2017**, *33*, 74–78. [CrossRef] [PubMed]
23. Chee, S.-P.; Chan, N.S.-W.; Yang, Y.; Ti, S.-E. Femtosecond laser-assisted cataract surgery for the white cataract. *Br. J. Ophthalmol.* **2018**, *103*, 544–550. [CrossRef]
24. Titiyal, J.S.; Kaur, M.; Falera, R. Intraoperative optical coherence tomography in anterior segment surgeries. *Indian J. Ophthalmol.* **2017**, *65*, 116–121. [CrossRef]
25. Pujari, A.; Sharma, N.; Bafna, R.K.; Agarwal, D. Study 3: Assessment of events during surgery on posterior polar cataracts using intraoperative optical coherence tomography. *Indian J. Ophthalmol.* **2021**, *69*, 594–597. [CrossRef]
26. Singh, A.; Vanathi, M.; Sahu, S.; Devi, S. Intraoperative OCT assisted descemetopexy with stromal vent incisions and intracameral gas injection for case of non-resolving Descemet's membrane detachment. *BMJ Case Rep.* **2017**, *2017*, 1–5. [CrossRef] [PubMed]
27. Sahay, P.; Shaji, K.R.; Maharana, P.K.; Titiyal, J.S. Spontaneous anterior dislocation of lens in a case of ectopia lentis et pupillae: A rare entity treated by a novel technique of microscope integrated optical coherence tomography (MIOCT) guided intralenticular lens aspiration. *BMJ Case Rep.* **2019**, *12*, 1–3. [CrossRef] [PubMed]

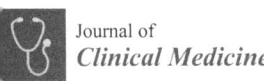

Journal of Clinical Medicine

Article

IOL Power Calculations and Cataract Surgery in Eyes with Previous Small Incision Lenticule Extraction

Roman Lischke [1], Walter Sekundo [2], Rainer Wiltfang [3,4], Martin Bechmann [3,4], Thomas C. Kreutzer [1], Siegfried G. Priglinger [1,5], Martin Dirisamer [1,5] and Nikolaus Luft [1,5,*]

[1] Department of Ophthalmology, University Hospital, Ludwig-Maximilians-University, 80337 Munich, Germany; r.lischke@campus.lmu.de (R.L.); thomas.kreutzer@med.uni-muenchen.de (T.C.K.); siegfried.priglinger@med.uni-muenchen.de (S.G.P.); martin.dirisamer@med.uni-muenchen.de (M.D.)
[2] SMILE Eyes Clinic, Department of Ophthalmology, Philipps University, 35043 Marburg, Germany; sekundo@med.uni-marburg.de
[3] SMILE Eyes Clinic, 85356 Munich, Germany; wiltfang@smileeyes.de (R.W.); bechmann@smileeyes.de (M.B.)
[4] SMILE Eyes Clinic, 54294 Trier, Germany
[5] SMILE Eyes Clinic, 4020 Linz, Austria
* Correspondence: nikolaus.luft@med.uni-muenchen.de; Tel.: +49-89-4400-53811; Fax: +49-89-4400-55160

Abstract: Small incision lenticule extraction (SMILE), with over 5 million procedures globally performed, will challenge ophthalmologists in the foreseeable future with accurate intraocular lens power calculations in an ageing population. After more than one decade since the introduction of SMILE, only one case report of cataract surgery with IOL implantation after SMILE is present in the peer-reviewed literature. Hence, the scope of the present multicenter study was to compare the IOL power calculation accuracy in post-SMILE eyes between ray tracing and a range of empirically optimized formulae available in the ASCRS post-keratorefractive surgery IOL power online calculator. In our study of 11 post-SMILE eyes undergoing cataract surgery, ray tracing showed the smallest mean absolute error (0.40 D) and yielded the largest percentage of eyes within ±0.50/±1.00 D (82/91%). The next best conventional formula was the Potvin–Hill formula with a mean absolute error of 0.66 D and an ±0.50/±1.00 D accuracy of 45 and 73%, respectively. Analyzing this first cohort of post-SMILE eyes undergoing cataract surgery and IOL implantation, ray tracing showed superior predictability in IOL power calculation over empirically optimized IOL power calculation formulae that were originally intended for use after Excimer-based keratorefractive procedures.

Keywords: SMILE; IOL calculation; ray tracing; cataract surgery

1. Introduction

Small incision lenticule extraction (SMILE), with over 5 million procedures performed globally, has evolved to one of the most popular and established keratorefractive procedures for the correction of myopia and myopic astigmatism. In the foreseeable future, the number of patients with prior SMILE treatment requiring cataract surgery is expected to increase accordingly in an ageing population. Inevitably, ophthalmologists will be challenged by accurate intraocular lens (IOL) power calculations for these patients.

There are three major problems in calculating IOL power after any kind of keratorefractive surgery. The first and most significant pitfall lies in the so-called keratometric index error [1]. In traditional keratometry, corneal radii are only measured for the anterior corneal curvature with the posterior corneal curvature radii being empirically extrapolated based on the assumption that the ratio between the anterior and posterior corneal curvature (A/P ratio) is constant, which is not the case after keratorefractive surgery. Secondly, some standard IOL calculation formulae tend to predict a more anterior effective lens position (formula error). Thirdly, the central zone of effective corneal power that had been artificially treated by keratorefractive surgery is estimated from traditional (paracentral) keratometry measurements. Therefore, the corneal power tends to be overestimated (instrument error) All these factors concordantly predispose to an underestimation in required IOL power and therefore lead to dissatisfying hyperopic residual refractive error after IOL implantation in eyes with prior myopic keratorefractive surgery [1].

Several methods have been introduced to address these sources of error and to reduce refractive surprises after keratorefractive surgery [2–9]. New technologies for corneal power measurements that incorporate measurements of the anterior and posterior corneal radii (e.g., total keratometry [10]) were established to enable more accurate predictions Moreover, sophisticated IOL power calculation formulae have been developed by means of empirical optimization; some of which consider pre-keratorefractive surgery data (Masket [11], Modfied-Masket or Barrett True-K formula), and some do not incorporate any preoperative values (Shammas [12], Barrett True-K no history, Potvin-Hill [13] or Haigis-L formula [14]). Conveniently, a range of these formulae is readily accessible in the American Society of Cataract and Refractive Surgeons (ASCRS) post-keratorefractive surgery IOL power online calculator.

In addition to these empirical formulae, the purely physical ray-tracing approach has demonstrated very good IOL power calculation outcomes in eyes with prior laser in situ keratomileusis (LASIK) or photorefractive keratectomy (PRK) [15–18]. The ray-tracing method measures the true shape of the cornea after corneal refractive surgery by using the anterior and posterior curvature radii and asphericity of these surfaces. Moreover, the central IOL thickness, the index of refraction and the true geometrical position, as defined by the ACD (distance between the posterior corneal apex and the anterior IOL apex), are used to describe the IOL and calculate its required power accurately. The ray-tracing method also obviates the need for any further historical or clinical data [5,15–17,19–21]. Ray tracing has been proven to provide reliable and satisfactory results in IOL calculations not only in treatment-naïve eyes but also in eyes after LASIK and PRK [15,16,18,21,22].

After more than one decade since the introduction of SMILE, only one case report of IOL calculation and implantation after SMILE is present in the peer-reviewed literature [23]. However, no formula comparison was reported. Hence, there is a deficiency in postoperative refractive data to optimize existing IOL power calculation formulae for post-SMILE eyes. In addition, corneal aberrometric changes after SMILE are significantly different when compared to the corneal shape changes after femtosecond laser-assisted LASIK (fs-LASIK) [24–26], which questions the validity of formulae optimized for Excimer-based photoablative procedures (e.g., the Masket formula) in post-SMILE eyes.

Consequently, the scope of the present multicenter study was to gather the first cohort of post-SMILE patients undergoing cataract extraction with IOL implantation. In this cohort, we set out to compare the refractive prediction error of IOL power calculations between ray tracing and various empirically optimized formulae available in the ASCRS post-keratorefractive surgery IOL power online calculator.

2. Materials and Methods

This multicenter cross-sectional study included patients that had previously undergone small incision lenticule extraction (SMILE) for the treatment of myopia and/or myopic astigmatism and later underwent cataract surgery with IOL implantation. The study was conducted at the University Eye Hospital of the Ludwig–Maximilians University (Munich, Germany), the SMILE Eyes Clinic Munich Airport (Munich, Germany) the SMILE Eyes Clinic Trier (Trier, Germany), the SMILE Eyes Center at the Department of Ophthalmology of the University of Marburg (Marburg, Germany) and the SMILE Eyes Clinic Linz (Linz, Austria).

Institutional review board approval of the Ludwig–Maximilians University Munich, was obtained for all aspects of this study; informed consent to use their data for analysis and publication was obtained from all subjects and all study-related procedures adhered to the tenets outlined in the The authors declare no conflict of interest.aration of Helsinki.

2.1. SMILE Surgery

All SMILE procedures were performed by highly experienced corneal surgeons utilizing the VisuMax 500-kHz femtosecond laser platform (Carl Zeiss Meditec AG, Jena, Germany) according to the local standards of the participating centers. The intended cap thickness was programmed at 120–130 μm with an intended optical zone size of 6.3 to 6.7 mm in diameter. At the superotemporal position, a single side cut of 50 degrees with a circumferential length of 3.0–4.0 mm was created. No intraoperative or postoperative complications were encountered. The surgical principles of the SMILE technique have been previously described in detail [27].

2.2. Cataract Surgery and IOL Implantation

Cataract surgery including IOL selection and implantation was performed by highly experienced corneal surgeons according to the local standards of the participating centers. Standard phacoemulsification with intracapsular IOL implantation was performed in all cases. A 2.5 mm clear incision at the steep corneal axis and two paracentesis incisions 2 clock hours away towards both directions were created. In case of a toric IOL, a clear corneal incision was created at the temporal corneal aspect. Cohesive and/or dispersive viscoelastic agents were used at the individual surgeon's discretion. No intraoperative or postoperative complications were encountered. The implanted IOL models and powers are summarized in Table 1.

Table 1. Implanted IOL models, powers and observed prediction errors.

Eye ID	Patient ID	Implanted IOL Model	Manufacturer	IOL Power (Spherical Equivalent, Diopters)	IOL-Power Calculation Formula Used	Prediction Error (Spherical Equivalent, Diopters)
1	1	CT Lucia 601PY	Carl Zeiss Meditec AG (Jena, Germany)	18.5	Haigis-L	0.68
2	1	CT Lucia 601PY	Carl Zeiss Meditec AG (Jena, Germany)	16.5	Haigis-L	−0.67
3	2	CT Lucia 601PY	Carl Zeiss Meditec AG (Jena, Germany)	21.0	Haigis-L	1.17
4	3	CT Lucia 611 PY	Carl Zeiss Meditec AG (Jena, Germany)	22.5	Haigis-L	−1.27
5	4	AcrySof IQ Toric SN6AT2/3	Alcon GmbH (Freiburg, Swiss)	25.0	Haigis-L	−0.51
6	4	AcrySof IQ Toric SN6AT2/3	Alcon GmbH (Freiburg, Swiss)	24.75	Haigis-L	−0.35
7	5	Lentis Comfort LS-313 MF15	Oculentis GmbH (Berlin, Germany)	21.0	Haigis-L	−0.84
8	5	Lentis Comfort LS-313 MF15	Oculentis GmbH (Berlin, Germany)	19.0	Haigis-L	−0.58
9	6	Polylens Y 50 P	Polytech-Domilens GmbH (Roßdorf, Germany)	19.5	Haigis-L	−3.76
10	6	Polylens Y 50 P	Polytech-Domilens GmbH (Roßdorf, Germany)	18.5	Haigis-L	−1.77
11	7	CT Asphina 409 MP	Carl Zeiss Meditec AG (Jena, Germany)	22.0	Ray tracing	−0.62

IOL, intraocular lens; D, diopter.

2.3. Subjective Refraction

Subjective manifest refraction was measured using the Jackson cross-cylinder method before and after each procedure. Best-corrected distance visual acuity (CDVA) was determined using standard ETDRS charts at 4 m.

2.4. Post-hoc IOL Power Calculation

Post-hoc IOL power calculation was performed utilizing dedicated-ray tracing software (Okulix; Panopsis, Mainz, Germany, Version 9.01) based on preoperative corneal tomography scans (Pentacam HR; Oculus Optikgeräte GmbH, Wetzlar, Germany), and preoperative optical biometry and anterior chamber depth measurements (IOLMaster 500 or 700; Carl Zeiss Meditec AG, Jena, Germany). Moreover, the American Society of Cataract and Refractive Surgery (ASCRS) post-keratorefractive surgery IOL power online calculator (Version 4.9; http://iolcalc.ascrs.org; last accessed on 4 October 2021) was used to calculate the predicted residual refractive error using the following formulae that consider pre-keratorefractive data: Barrett True K, Masket [11] and Modified Masket. Additionally, the following formulae available in the ASCRS calculator were used, which do not incorporate preoperative data: Barrett True K No History, Haigis-L [14], Potvin-Hill [13] and Shammas [12]. In accordance with recent recommendations for IOL power calculation studies [28], no IOL constant optimization was performed but (when appropriate) optimized IOL constants were used as published on the User Group for Laser Interference Biometry (ULIB) website (http://ocusoft.de/ulib/index.htm; last accessed on 4 October 2021).

2.5. Statistical Analysis

On the basis of established protocols for studies on IOL power calculation formula accuracy [28,29], the prediction error (PE) was defined as the difference between the actual residual refraction and the residual refraction predicted by the respective IOL power calculation method for the same IOL power and model. The arithmetic mean of the PE was referred to as the mean error (ME). Moreover, all negative errors were converted to positive to calculate the mean absolute error (MAE) as well as the median absolute error (MedAE). Furthermore, the standard deviation, minimum and maximum (range of PE) as well as the percentage of eyes within ±0.50, ±1.00, ±1.50 and ±2.00 diopter (D) are reported [28,29]. Boxplots were created to illustrate the differences in PE between different IOL power calculation formulae. Normal distribution was tested by the Shapiro–Wilk method. The Kruskal–Wallis test was employed to assess the differences in PE between formulae and ray tracing. In addition, the variance of ME was calculated—a smaller variance indicates better consistency of a IOL calculation method [30]. The Fisher's exact test with the Bonferroni correction was used to test for statistically significant differences between proportions of eyes with PEs within ±0.50 D and ±1.00 D, respectively., A p-value of <0.05 was defined as being indicative of statistical significance. All statistical analyses were performed using SPSS 27.0.0.0 for Windows (IBM Corp.; Armonk, NY, USA).

3. Results

A total of 11 eyes of 7 patients [1 (14%) female] were included with a mean follow up after SMILE of 2 ± 1 months (range of 1 to 4 months) and a mean follow up after cataract surgery of 8 ± 11 months (range of 1 to 38 months). The mean period of time between SMILE and cataract procedures were 31 ± 16 months (range 12 to 54 months). Subjects' baseline characteristics are summarized in Table 2. The mean pre- and post SMILE manifest refraction spherical equivalent (SE) was −5.15 ± 1.31 diopters (D; range −7.00 to −3.00 D) and −0.48 ± 0.57 D (range: −1.63 to +0.38 D), respectively. The mean preoperative SE before cataract surgery was −2.44 ± 2.48 D (range: −7.63 to +0.63 D). One patient developed a nuclear cataract, which lead to an index myopia of −7.63 D of SE. After cataract surgery, the mean SE amounted to −0.68 ± 0.65 D (range: −2.00 to 0.00 D).

Table 2. Subjects' characteristics.

	Parameter	Mean	Median	SD	Range
	Age at SMILE (years)	46.43	46	6.75	37 to 55
	Age at cataract surgery (years)	49.45	49	7.31	38 to 59
SMILE	Preoperative Manifest Refraction (D)				
	Sphere	−4.86	−5.25	1.30	−6.50 to −2.75
	Cylinder	−0.57	−0.50	0.23	−1.00 to −0.25
	Spherical Equivalent	−5.15	−5.38	1.31	−7.00 to −3.00
	Postoperative Manifest Refraction (D)				
	Sphere	−0.34	−0.5	0.5	−1.75 to 0.50
	Cylinder	−0.27	−0.25	0.24	−0.75 to 0.00
	Spherical Equivalent	−0.48	−0.50	0.57	−1.63 to 0.38
Cataract surgery	Preoperative Manifest Refraction (D)				
	Sphere	−2.00	−1.5	2.49	−7.00 to 1.25
	Cylinder	−0.89	−1.00	0.58	−2.00 to −0.25
	Spherical Equivalent	−2.44	−2.25	2.48	−7.63 to 0.63
	Postoperative Manifest Refraction (D)				
	Sphere	−0.45	0.00	0.72	−2.00 to 0.25
	Cylinder	−0.45	−0.5	0.4	−1.25 to 0.00
	Spherical Equivalent	−0.68	−0.63	0.65	−2.00 to 0.00

SD, standard deviation; D, diopter; SMILE, small incision lenticle extraction; BCVA, best corrected visual acuity.

The performance of the investigated IOL power calculation formulae in reference to physical ray tracing is summarized in Table 3 and visualized by boxplots (Figure 1). On average, the formulae concordantly overestimated the required IOL power. Of all investigated traditional formulae, the Potvin–Hill formula yielded the smallest ME (−0.06 ± 0.86 D, range −1.67 to 1.22) and the Shammas formula resulted in the largest IOL power overestimation with a ME of −0.96 ± 1.14 D (range −2.32 to 1.07). Ray tracing was the only method resulting in a hyperopic ME of 0.18 D ± 0.48 D (range −0.43 to 1.22), even though in absolute terms the ME was the lowest (Table 3). Nevertheless, Kruskal–Wallis testing revealed no statistically significant differences in ME between the different IOL power calculation methods (p = 0.16).

Table 3. Formula performance in comparison.

	Formula	Prediction Error (D)				Absolute Error (D)		% of Eyes within PE Range Indicated			
		Mean	SD	Range	Variance (D²)	Mean	Median	±0.5 D	±1.0 D	±1.5 D	±2.0 D
	Ray tracing	0.18	0.48	−0.43 to 1.22	0.23	0.4	0.36	82	91	100	100
Using prior data	Masket	−0.25	0.98	−1.99 to 1.4	0.95	0.81	0.82	36	64	91	100
	Modified-Masket	−0.55	0.91	−2.23 to 0.94	0.83	0.85	0.67	27	64	91	91
	Barret True-K	−0.27	0.98	−2.32 to 1.07	0.96	0.80	0.72	27	73	91	91
	Shammas	−0.96	1.14	−2.53 to 0.67	1.3	1.14	0.94	27	55	73	91
Using no prior data	Haigis-L	−0.81	1.28	−3.76 to 1.17	1.63	1.14	0.84	9	64	82	91
	Potvin-Hill	−0.06	0.86	−1.67 to 1.22	0.74	0.66	0.52	45	73	91	100
	Barrett True K no history	−0.44	1.13	−2.90 to 1.12	1.27	0.93	0.67	27	73	91	91

D, diopters; PE, prediction error; SD, standard deviation.

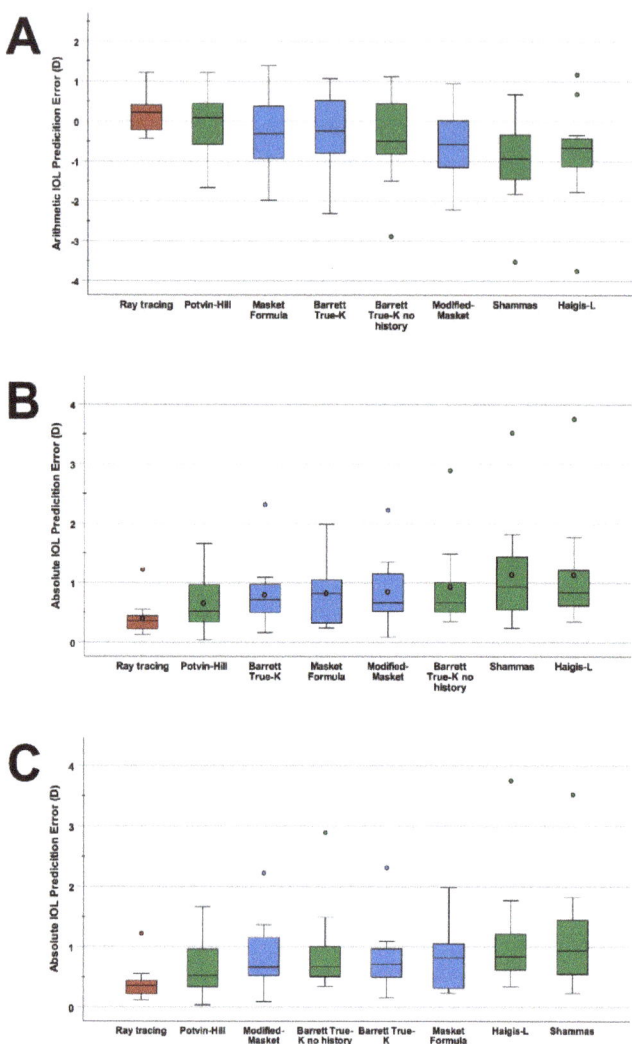

Figure 1. Prediction errors of IOL power calculation formulae. Blue boxplots show formulae that incorporate clinical history data and green boxplots show formulae that do not use any prior keratorefractive surgery data. The red boxplots represent ray tracing. (**A**) IOL power calculation formulae ranked from left to right according to their arithmetic prediction errors. (**B**) IOL power calculation formulae ranked from left to right according to their MAE. Circles demonstrate the respective MAE of each formula. (**C**) IOL power calculation formulae ranked from left to right according to their MedAE. (D, diopter).

With respect to MAE and MedAE, ray tracing achieved the smallest MAE (0.40 D) and MedAE (0.36 D) of all examined methods. Of the various tested formulae from the ASCRS calculator, the Potvin–Hill formula yield the smallest MAE (0.66 D), closely followed by the Barrett True-K (0.80 D) and the Masket formula (0.81 D). The Potvin–Hill formula also yielded the smallest MedAE (0.52 D) of all conventional IOL formulae. Kruskal–Wallis testing, however, revealed no statistically significant differences in MAE ($p = 0.085$) and on MedAE ($p = 0.095$). Regarding the variance of ME, the ray-tracing method showed the smallest variance (0.23 D^2), followed by the Potvin–Hill (0.74 D^2) and Modified Masket (0.83 D^2) formulae. The Haigis-L formula showed the highest variance (1.63 D^2).

With 82%, the ray-tracing method yielded the highest percentage of eyes within a refractive prediction error of ±0.50 D (Figure 2). The next best conventional formula was the Potvin–Hill formula with an ±0.50 D accuracy of 45%. The Haigis-L formula showed the lowest ±0.50 D accuracy of 9%. The Fisher's exact test indicated significant differences between proportions of eyes with PEs of ±0.50 D (p = 0.034). The Bonferroni correction was employed to investigate these differences in detail, showing statistically significant differences between the ray-tracing method and each of the conventional IOL power calculation formulae (all with $p < 0.001$). No statistically significant differences could be found in the proportions of eyes with PEs of ±1.00 D (p = 0.754). Nevertheless, the ray-tracing method achieved the highest ±1.00 D accuracy (91%), followed by the Potvin–Hill, Barrett True-K and Barrett True-K no history formulae (all 73%). The Shammas formula showed the lowest ±1.00 D accuracy of 55%.

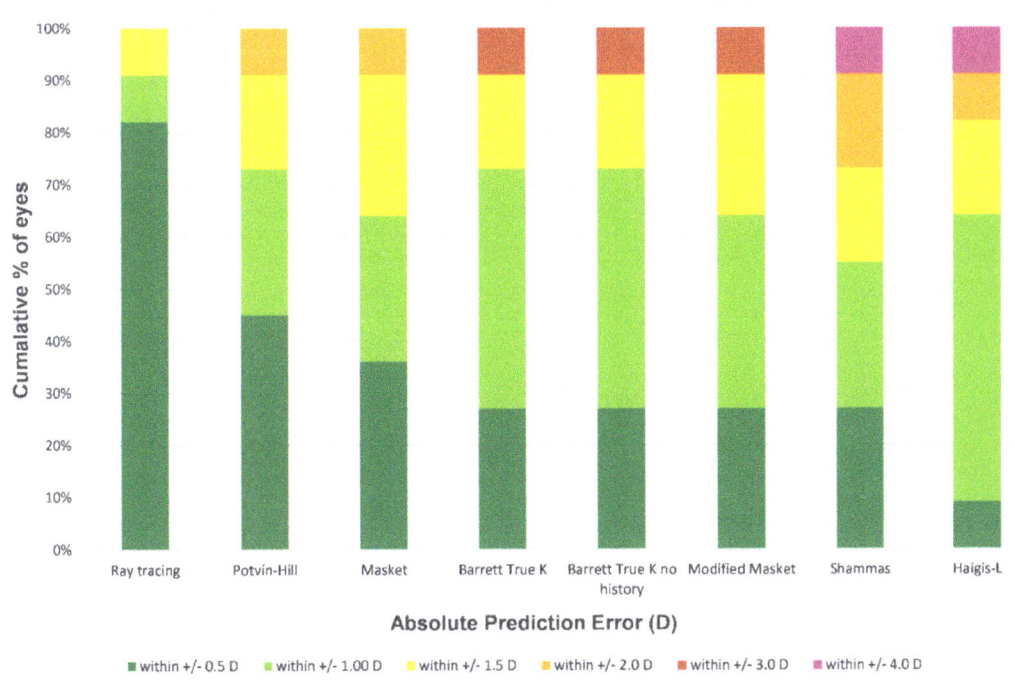

Figure 2. Histogram analysis comparing the percentage of eyes within given prediction error ranges. The formulas were sorted by the proportion of eyes within ±0.50 D in descending order.

4. Discussion

In this first study of its kind, ray tracing was compared to six established IOL power calculation formulae available in the ASCRS online calculator in post-SMILE eyes undergoing cataract surgery. In our analysis, the ray tracing method showed the most accurate IOL power calculation with a ME of 0.18 ± 0.48 D and 82% of eyes being within ±0.50 D and 91% of eyes within ±1.00 D.

Our findings endorse previous, purely theoretical studies (with no actually performed cataract surgery) in eyes after SMILE. Lazaridis et al. [31] used a theoretical model including virtual IOL implantation to evaluate prediction errors between ray tracing and four conventional IOL power calculation formulae. In their analysis, ray tracing yielded the smallest ME of −0.06 ± 0.40 D and a PE of ±0.5 D in 81.9% of eyes, which is highly coherent with our findings after actual cataract surgery. Moreover, the lowest ME variance (as an indicator of the consistency of an IOL power calculation method), was achieved by ray tracing in both studies. Interestingly, Lazaridis et al. [31] reported better results for the Haigis-L formula (ME of −0.39 ± 0.62 D and 53.4% of eyes with PEs within ± 0.5 D) as compared to our "real world" analysis, where Haigis-L yielded the worst ±0.50 D accuracy of only 9% of all investigated formulae and a ME of −0.81 ± 1.28 D.

In the second previous theoretical study, our group [32] compared the predicted postoperative residual refractive error of the IOL determined by ray tracing with the residual refraction of the same IOL as predicted by a range of conventional IOL power calculation formulae available in the ASCRS post-keratorefractive surgery IOL power calculator. The Masket formula showed the smallest ME (−0.36 ± 0.32 D) and yielded the largest percentage of eyes within ±0.50 D (70%) in reference to the prediction of ray tracing which was defined as the gold standard method for the purpose of that study. Non-inferior MEs and ±0.50 D accuracies were achieved by the Barrett True K, Barrett True K no history and the Potvin–Hill formula [32].

In the third purely theoretical study, Zhu et al. [33] used the concept of equivalent IOL power differences (EILD) as an indicator for the "stability" of four conventional IOL calculation formulae in post-SMILE eyes. The Barrett True-K and Haigis formulae showed similar stability in eyes with axial lengths between 24 and 26 mm (85.19 vs. 88.89% for a margin of error within 0.5 D; 100 vs. 100% for a margin of error within 1.0 D). In eyes with an axial length of >26 mm, the Barrett True-K formula was the most "stable" formula with respective percentages of 81.49 and 92.59% for margin errors within 0.5 and 1.0 D, respectively.

These compiled theoretical data are confirmed by the present "real world" study, in which the Potvin–Hill and Masket formula showed the best PEs of all conventional formulae. The Potvin–Hill formula yielded the best ME in the present study (ME −0.06 ± 0.86 D and 45% of eyes within ±0.50 D) closely followed by ray tracing (ME 0.18 ± 0.48 D and 82% of eyes within ±0.50 D) and the Masket formula (ME −0.25 ± 0.98 D and 36% of eyes within ±0.50 D). Moreover, the accuracy of the Barrett True K formula was non-inferior when preoperative refractive data were not entered but estimated with the Barrett True K no history formula. By using adjusted keratometry readings, the Shammas formula showed the greatest overestimation of IOL power of all the investigated formulae. Highly congruent findings were also made in the previous theoretical study of our group [32].

As a purely physical approach based on Snell's law, ray tracing offers many advantages over conventional IOL power calculation formulae in post-keratorefractive surgery eyes. Unlike empirically optimized regression formulae, ray tracing does not rely on any fictional keratometric index or "fudge factors" but utilizes measurements of both the anterior and posterior corneal radii to determine total corneal power. Hence, the need for any empirical optimization, clinical history or preoperative refractive data is obsolete. The latter can be a pivotal advantage in eyes with index myopia due to cataract formation and unknown post-keratorefractive surgery refraction.

These theoretical methodological advantages of the ray tracing principle have been previously proven in different samples of post-Excimer ablation eyes undergoing cataract surgery with IOL implantation [15,16,18]. For instance, Savini et al. [16] yielded 71.4% of 21 post myopic Excimer ablation eyes within ± 0.50 D and 85.7% within ± 1.00 D of the predicted refraction utilizing ray tracing. These results seem comparable to our findings in post-SMILE eyes. Saiki et al. [18] reported slightly subpar outcomes for ray tracing in their sample of 24 post myopic LASIK eyes with ±0.50 D and ±1.00 accuracies of 42 and 75%, respectively. Furthermore, the arithmetic prediction error of ray tracing of 0.63 ± 0.85 D indicated an underestimation of IOL power entailing unpleasant hyperopic residual refractive errors after cataract surgery. In our study, we also observed a minimal hyperopic ME for ray tracing after SMILE, even though it was more than three times smaller (0.18 ± 0.48 D).

First recommendations for clinicians encountering post myopic SMILE patients requiring cataract surgery can be formulated based on the findings of the present study. Physical ray tracing should be employed for IOL power calculation and surgeons should be aware of a slight hyperopic ME of less than +0.25 D when selecting the appropriate IOL power, which is only available in 0.50 D steps for most contemporary IOL models. Ray tracing calculations should ideally be interpreted in conjunction with the Potvin-Hill and Masket formula, which should provide comparable results.

Limitations to this study might be found. First and foremost, the study is limited by its relatively small sample size. Nevertheless, the present work represents the first cohort of post-SMILE patients undergoing cataract surgery and may provide clinicians important guidance for IOL power selection. The paucity of post-SMILE cataract cases in Austria and Germany, where the SMILE technique was developed and first introduced more than a decade ago, also prompted us to include both eyes of some patients into the analysis. For the same reason and due to the multicenter approach, the authors felt inclined to accept multiple IOL types, surgeons and surgical protocols. A further limitation of the present study is that not all formulae currently available in the ASCRS calculator could be included as no Atlas-, Galilei- or OCT-based corneal measurements were available.

In summary, this study comprises the first cohort of post myopic SMILE eyes undergoing cataract surgery and IOL implantation. In post-SMILE eyes, ray tracing facilitated IOL power calculations with a superior accuracy and should be the first choice over conventional IOL power calculation formulae that are empirically optimized for post-Excimer ablation eyes.

Author Contributions: Conceptualization, R.L. and N.L.; methodology, R.L. and N.L.; validation, R.L., W.S., R.W., M.B., T.C.K., S.G.P., M.D. and N.L.; formal analysis, R.L., W.S., R.W., M.B., T.C.K., S.G.P., M.D. and N.L.; investigation, R.L., W.S., R.W., M.B., T.C.K., S.G.P., M.D. and N.L.; resources, R.L., W.S., R.W., M.B., T.C.K., S.G.P., M.D. and N.L.; data curation, R.L., W.S., R.W., M.B., T.C.K., S.G.P., M.D. and N.L.; writing—original draft preparation, R.L.; writing—review and editing, R.L. and N.L.; visualization, R.L.; supervision, N.L.; project administration, N.L. All authors have read and agreed to the published version of the manuscript.

Funding: This research received no external funding.

Institutional Review Board Statement: The study was conducted in accordance with the Declaration of Helsinki and approved by the local institutional review board of the Ludwig Maximilian University for studies involving humans.

Informed Consent Statement: Informed consent was obtained from all subjects involved in the study.

Data Availability Statement: The datasets used and analyzed during the current study are available from the corresponding author on reasonable request.

Conflicts of Interest: The authors declare no conflict of interest.

References

1. Hoffer, K.J. Intraocular lens power calculation after previous laser refractive surgery. *J. Cataract. Refract. Surg.* **2009**, *354*, 759–765. [CrossRef] [PubMed]
2. Wang, L.; Booth, M.A.; Koch, D.D. Comparison of intraocular lens power calculation methods in eyes that have undergone LASIK. *Ophthalmology* **2004**, *11110*, 1825–1831. [CrossRef] [PubMed]
3. Mackool, R.J.; Ko, W.; Mackool, R. Intraocular lens power calculation after laser in situ keratomileusis: Aphakic refraction technique. *J. Cataract Refract. Surg.* **2006**, *323*, 435–437. [CrossRef] [PubMed]
4. Borasio, E.; Stevens, J.; Smith, G.T. Estimation of true corneal power after keratorefractive surgery in eyes requiring cataract surgery: BESSt formula. *J. Cataract Refract. Surg.* **2006**, *3212*, 2004–2014. [CrossRef]
5. Jin, H.; Rabsilber, T.; Ehmer, A.; Borkenstein, A.F.; Limberger, I.-J.; Guo, H.; Auffarth, G.U. Comparison of ray-tracing method and thin-lens formula in intraocular lens power calculations. *J. Cataract Refract. Surg.* **2009**, *354*, 650–662. [CrossRef]
6. Abulafia, A.; Hill, W.E.; Koch, D.D.; Wang, L.; Barrett, G.D. Accuracy of the Barrett True-K formula for intraocular lens power prediction after laser in situ keratomileusis or photorefractive keratectomy for myopia. *J. Cataract Refract. Surg.* **2016**, *423*, 363–369. [CrossRef]

7. Wang, L.; Tang, M.; Huang, D.; Weikert, M.P.; Koch, D.D. Comparison of Newer Intraocular Lens Power Calculation Methods for Eyes after Corneal Refractive Surgery. *Ophthalmology* **2015**, *12212*, 2443–2449. [CrossRef]
8. Fram, N.R.; Masket, S.; Wang, L. Comparison of Intraoperative Aberrometry, OCT-Based IOL Formula, Haigis-L, and Masket Formulae for IOL Power Calculation after Laser Vision Correction. *Ophthalmology* **2015**, *1226*, 1096–1101. [CrossRef]
9. Canto, A.P.; Chhadva, P.; Cabot, F.; Galor, A.; Yoo, S.H.; Vaddavalli, P.K.; Culbertson, W.W. Comparison of IOL power calculation methods and intraoperative wavefront aberrometer in eyes after refractive surgery. *J. Refract. Surg.* **2013**, *297*, 484–489. [CrossRef]
10. Lischke, R.; Mayer, W.J.; Feucht, N.; Siedlecki, J.; Wiltfang, R.; Kook, D.; Priglinger, S.G.; Luft, N. Total keratometry for determination of true corneal power after myopic small-incision lenticule extraction. *J. Cataract Refract. Surg.* **2021**, *4710*, 1285–1289. [CrossRef]
11. Masket, S.; Masket, S.E. Simple regression formula for intraocular lens power adjustment in eyes requiring cataract surgery after excimer laser photoablation. *J. Cataract Refract. Surg.* **2006**, *323*, 430–434. [CrossRef]
12. Shammas, H.J.; Shammas, M.C. No-history method of intraocular lens power calculation for cataract surgery after myopic laser in situ keratomileusis. *J. Cataract Refract. Surg.* **2007**, *331*, 31–36. [CrossRef]
13. Potvin, R.; Hill, W. New algorithm for intraocular lens power calculations after myopic laser in situ keratomileusis based on rotating Scheimpflug camera data. *J. Cataract Refract. Surg.* **2015**, *412*, 339–347. [CrossRef]
14. Haigis, W. Intraocular lens calculation after refractive surgery for myopia: Haigis-L formula. *J. Cataract Refract. Surg.* **2008**, *3410*, 1658–1663. [CrossRef]
15. Rabsilber, T.M.; Reuland, A.J.; Holzer, M.P.; Auffarth, G.U. Intraocular lens power calculation using ray tracing following excimer laser surgery. *Eye* **2007**, *216*, 697–701. [CrossRef]
16. Savini, G.; Bedei, A.; Barboni, P.; Ducoli, P.; Hoffer, K.J. Intraocular lens power calculation by ray-tracing after myopic excimer laser surgery. *Am. J. Ophthalmol.* **2014**, *1571*, 150–153.e151. [CrossRef]
17. Savini, G.; Calossi, A.; Camellin, M.; Carones, F.; Fantozzi, M.; Hoffer, K.J. Corneal ray tracing versus simulated keratometry for estimating corneal power changes after excimer laser surgery. *J. Cataract Refract. Surg.* **2014**, *407*, 1109–1115. [CrossRef]
18. Saiki, M.; Negishi, K.; Kato, N.; Torii, H.; Dogru, M.; Tsubota, K. Ray tracing software for intraocular lens power calculation after corneal excimer laser surgery. *Jpn J. Ophthalmol.* **2014**, *583*, 276–281. [CrossRef]
19. Preussner, P.R.; Wahl, J.; Lahdo, H.; Dick, B.; Findl, O. Ray tracing for intraocular lens calculation. *J. Cataract Refract. Surg.* **2002**, *288*, 1412–1419. [CrossRef]
20. Canovas, C.; van der Mooren, M.; Rosén, R.; Piers, P.A.; Wang, L.; Koch, D.D.; Artal, P. Effect of the equivalent refractive index on intraocular lens power prediction with ray tracing after myopic laser in situ keratomileusis. *J. Cataract Refract. Surg.* **2015**, *415*, 1030–1037. [CrossRef]
21. Hoffmann, P.; Wahl, J.; Preussner, P.R. Accuracy of intraocular lens calculation with ray tracing. *J. Refract. Surg.* **2012**, *289*, 650–655. [CrossRef] [PubMed]
22. Ghoreyshi, M.; Khalilian, A.; Peyman, M.; Mohammadinia, M.; Peyman, A. Comparison of OKULIX ray-tracing software with SRK-T and Hoffer-Q formula in intraocular lens power calculation. *J. Curr. Ophthalmol.* **2018**, *301*, 63–67. [CrossRef] [PubMed]
23. Ganesh, S.; Brar, S.; Sriprakash, K. Post-small incision lenticule extraction phacoemulsification with multifocal IOL implantation: A case report. *Indian J. Ophthalmol.* **2019**, *678*, 1353–1356.
24. Gyldenkerne, A.; Ivarsen, A.; Hjortdal, J. Comparison of corneal shape changes and aberrations induced By FS-LASIK and SMILE for myopia. *J. Refract. Surg.* **2015**, *314*, 223–229. [CrossRef]
25. Lazaridis, A.; Spiru, B.; Giallouros, E.; Droutsas, K.; Messerschmidt-Roth, A.; Sekundo, W. Corneal Remodeling After Myopic SMILE Versus FS-LASIK. *Cornea* **2021**, *41*, 826–832. [CrossRef]
26. Zhang, Y.L.; Cao, L.J.; Chen, H.W.; Xu, X.H.; Li, Z.N.; Liu, L. Comparison of changes in refractive error and corneal curvature following small-incision lenticule extraction and femtosecond laser-assisted in situ keratomileusis surgery. *Indian J. Ophthalmol.* **2018**, *66*, 1562–1567. [CrossRef]
27. Sekundo, W.; Kunert, K.S.; Blum, M. Small incision corneal refractive surgery using the small incision lenticule extraction (SMILE) procedure for the correction of myopia and myopic astigmatism: Results of a 6 month prospective study. *Br. J. Ophthalmol.* **2011**, *953*, 335–339. [CrossRef]
28. Hoffer, K.J.; Savini, G. Update on Intraocular Lens Power Calculation Study Protocols: The Better Way to Design and Report Clinical Trials. *Ophthalmology* **2021**, *12811*, e115–e120. [CrossRef]
29. Hoffer, K.J.; Aramberri, J.; Haigis, W.; Olsen, T.; Savini, G.; Shammas, H.J.; Bentow, S. Protocols for studies of intraocular lens formula accuracy. *Am. J. Ophthalmol.* **2015**, *1603*, 403–405.e401. [CrossRef]
30. Patel, P.; Ashena, Z.; Vasavada, V.; Vasavada, S.; Vasavada, V.; Sudhalkar, A.; Nanavaty, M. Comparison of intraocular lens calculation methods after myopic laser-assisted in situ keratomileusis and radial keratotomy without prior refractive data. *Br. J. Ophthalmol.* **2020**, *106*, 47–53. [CrossRef]
31. Lazaridis, A.; Schraml, F.; Preussner, P.R.; Sekundo, W. Predictability of intraocular lens power calculation after small-incision lenticule extraction for myopia. *J. Cataract Refract. Surg.* **2021**, *473*, 304–310. [CrossRef]
32. Luft, N.; Siedlecki, J.; Schworm, B.; Kreutzer, T.C.; Mayer, W.J.; Priglinger, S.G.; Dirisamer, M. Intraocular Lens Power Calculation after Small Incision Lenticule Extraction. *Sci. Rep.* **2020**, *101*, 5982. [CrossRef]
33. Zhu, W.; Zhang, F.J.; Li, Y.; Song, Y.Z. Stability of the Barrett True-K formula for intraocular lens power calculation after SMILE in Chinese myopic eyes. *Int. J. Ophthalmol.* **2020**, *134*, 560–566. [CrossRef]

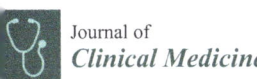

Article

Investigating the Prediction Accuracy of Recently Updated Intraocular Lens Power Formulas with Artificial Intelligence for High Myopia

Miki Omoto, Kaoruko Sugawara, Hidemasa Torii, Erisa Yotsukura, Sachiko Masui, Yuta Shigeno, Yasuyo Nishi and Kazuno Negishi *

Department of Ophthalmology, Keio University School of Medicine, Tokyo 160-8582, Japan
* Correspondence: kazunonegishi@keio.jp; Tel.: +81-3-3353-1211

Abstract: The aim of this study was to investigate the prediction accuracy of intraocular lens (IOL) power formulas with artificial intelligence (AI) for high myopia. Cases of highly myopic patients (axial length [AL], >26.0 mm) undergoing uncomplicated cataract surgery with at least 1-month follow-up were included. Prediction errors, absolute errors, and percentages of eyes with prediction errors within ±0.25, ±0.50, and ±1.00 diopters (D) were compared using five formulas: Hill-RBF3.0, Kane, Barrett Universal II (BUII), Haigis, and SRK/T. Seventy eyes (mean patient age at surgery, 64.0 ± 9.0 years; mean AL, 27.8 ± 1.3 mm) were included. The prediction errors with the Hill-RBF3.0 and Kane formulas were statistically different from the BUII, Haigis, and SRK/T formulas, whereas there was not a statistically significant difference between those with the Hill-RBF3.0 and Kane. The absolute errors with the Hill-RBF3.0 and Kane formulas were smaller than that with the BUII formula, whereas there was not a statistically significant difference between the other formulas. The percentage within ±0.25 D with the Hill-RBF3.0 formula was larger than that with the BUII formula. The prediction accuracy using AI (Hill-RBF3.0 and Kane) showed excellent prediction accuracy. No significant difference was observed in the prediction accuracy between the Hill-RBF3.0 and Kane formulas.

Keywords: cataract; intraocular lens; artificial intelligence

1. Introduction

The primary purpose of cataract surgery is visual rehabilitation; however, refractive correction is also an important aspect of the surgery to achieve better vision and quality of life postoperatively. With modern surgical techniques, patients' expectations for better vision postoperatively are increasing day by day. Accurately predicting the postoperative refraction in myopic eyes is challenging [1,2]. The prevalence of myopia is growing, especially in Asia [3–5]. While many methods are being used to overcome this issue [6–11], the challenge still remains.

The recent advances in artificial intelligence (AI) are outstanding and the application of AI in clinical medicine is a current hot topic. AI is used not only for classification or anomaly detection, but also for regression. The Hill-RBF refractive formula uses pattern recognition and data interpolation to predict postoperative refraction [12,13], whereas the Kane formula is based on theoretical optics and also incorporates regression and AI components to further refine its predictions [14]. Several studies have reported good refractive outcomes obtained with these formulas [15–17].

The Hill-RBF formula has been updated recently to version 3.0, which was reported to show better prediction accuracy than the previous version in a recent study; however, that study did not focus on myopic eyes (axial length [AL], 24.10 ± 1.47 mm) [13] and, to our knowledge, no other study has investigated the accuracy of the new version of the formula

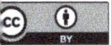

in myopic eyes. Therefore, we investigated the prediction accuracy of the recently updated intraocular lens (IOL) power formulas with AI for high myopia.

2. Materials and Methods

2.1. Study Institutions and Institutional Review Board Approval

The Research Ethics Committee of the Graduate School of Medicine and the Faculty of Medicine at Keio University approved this retrospective, observational study. All patients provided written consent for the surgeries. Patient consent to participate in this study was waived, and an opt-out approach was used according to the Ethical Guidelines for Medical and Health Research Involving Human Subjects presented by the Ministry of Education, Culture, Sports, Science, and Technology in Japan. The patients and public were not involved in the design, conduct, reporting, or dissemination plans of our research. This study was performed according to the tenets of the Declaration of Helsinki.

2.2. Participants

The study participants were retrospectively recruited at the institution. Cases of uncomplicated cataract surgery for highly myopic eyes (AL > 26.0 mm) with at least 1 month postoperative follow-up were included. Eyes with a vision-affecting ocular disease other than cataract or that had undergone past refractive surgeries were excluded. When both eyes of a patient met the criteria, we randomly selected one eye for inclusion. Seventy eyes of seventy patients were included in the final analysis. One surgeon (NK) performed all surgeries. Phacoemulsification and intraocular lens (IOL) implantation were performed through a 2.4 mm sutureless corneal incision. The implanted IOL was the TECNIS® Monofocal (clear ZCB00) in 28 eyes or the yellow-tinted lens (ZCB00V) in 42 eyes (both from Johnson & Johnson, Santa Ana, CA, USA).

2.3. IOL Power Calculation

All patients underwent biometric measurements using the IOLMaster® 700 (Carl Zeiss Meditec AG, Jena, Germany) preoperatively. Using the parameters, the postoperative refraction was predicted using five formulas: Hill-RBF3.0, Kane, Barrett Universal II (BUII), Haigis, and SRK/T. The Hill-RBF Calculator is an advanced, self-validating method for IOL power selection employing pattern recognition and a sophisticated form of data interpolation that can be used with other biconvex IOL models in the power range of +6.00 to +30.00 D and other meniscus IOL designs from −5.00 to +5.00 D [12,13]. The Kane formula is based on theoretical optics and incorporates both regression and artificial intelligence components to further refine its predictions [14]. BUII is a Gaussian-based formula for thick lenses using paraxial ray tracing, which takes into account changes in the principal plane that occur with various IOL powers, but the details are not disclosed. Hiagis and SRK/T are theoretical formulas for predicting effective lens position based on the multiple regression of the A constant, anterior chamber depth, and axial length in Haigis and the corneal curvature radius and axial length in SRK/T, respectively. The Wang Koch (WK) axial length adjustment was applied for these two formulas. [2,11,18,19]. The lens constants were set as 119.30 for the Hill-RBF3, BUII, and SRK/T formulas; 119.36 for the Kane formula; and −1.302 (A0), 0.210 (A1), and 0.251 (A2) for the Haigis formula.

2.4. Statistical Analysis

The best-corrected visual acuity (BCVA) measurements were performed 1 month postoperatively. First, the prediction error was calculated by subtracting the predicted value with the implanted IOL from the postoperative subjective spherical equivalent. The absolute error was then calculated as the absolute value of the prediction error. The percentages of eyes with a prediction error of ±0.25, ±0.50, and ±1.00 D were also calculated for each formula. The prediction and absolute errors were compared among the formulas using the Friedman test, followed by post hoc analysis using the pairwise Wilcoxon signed-rank test with Bonferroni correction. The percentages were compared using Cochran's Q test followed by post hoc analysis using the McNemar test with Bonferroni correction. Subanalyses were also performed in each of the following subgroups: eyes with an AL > 28.0 mm and eyes with an AL < 28.0 mm. Statistical significance was $p < 0.05$. All analyses were performed using R software v.4.0.4 (The R Foundation for Statistical Computing, Vienna, Austria).

3. Results

The demographic data of the 70 study eyes are summarized in Table 1. The mean ± standard deviation (SD) age at the time of surgery was 64.0 ± 9.0 years. The mean ± SD AL preoperatively was 27.8 ± 1.3 mm. Forty-five eyes had an AL < 28.0 mm and twenty-five eyes had an AL > 28.0 mm.

Table 1. Demographics of the study subjects.

Variables	Values
Number of eyes	70 eyes of 70 patients
Right/left	33/37
Male/female	38/32
Age at the surgery (years)	64.0 ± 9.0
Best corrected visual acuity (logMAR)	0.14 ± 0.26
Spherical equivalent (D)	−9.73 ± 4.40
Target refraction (D)	−1.79 ± 1.15
Axial length (mm)	27.84 ± 1.34
Keratometry (D)	54.3 ± 24.9
Anterior chamber depth (mm)	3.45 ± 0.35
Lens thickness (mm)	4.45 ± 0.37
Central corneal thickness (μm)	556 ± 38

logMAR = logarithm of the minimum angle of resolution; D = diopters.

Figure 1A shows the prediction error with each formula. The values with the Hill-RBF3.0 and Kane formulas were statistically different from the BUII, Haigis, and SRK/T formulas, whereas there was not a statistically significant difference between those with the Hill-RBF3.0 and Kane formula (Tables 2 and S1).

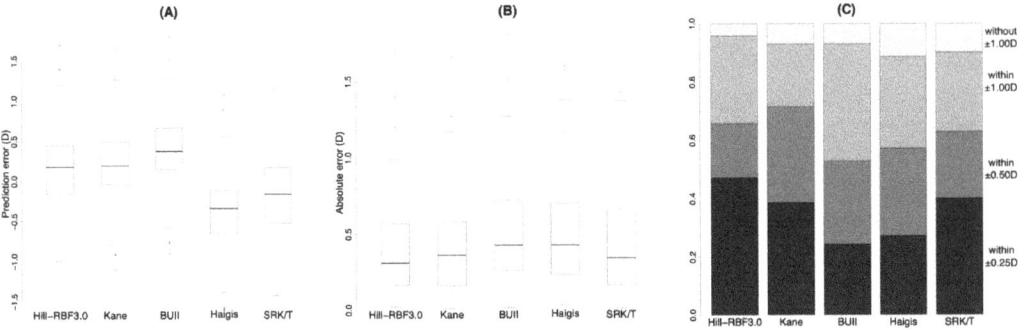

Figure 1. Prediction error (**A**), absolute error (**B**) and stacked bar chart (**C**) of prediction accuracy with each formula. BUII = Barrett Universal II; D = diopters. Wang Koch adjustment was applied for the Haigis and SRK/T formulas.

Table 2. Prediction accuracy with each formula.

		Hill-RBF3.0	Kane	BUII	Haigis	SRK/T	p-Value
Prediction error (D)	Mean ± SD	0.17 ± 0.52	0.19 ± 0.51	0.36 ± 0.51	−0.38 ± 0.52	−0.18 ± 0.58	<0.001 *
	Median	0.18	0.2	0.38 [†,‡]	−0.34 [†,‡,§]	−0.16 [†,‡,§,∥]	
Absolute error (D)	Mean ± SD	0.42 ± 0.34	0.42 ± 0.34	0.51 ± 0.35	0.52 ± 0.38	0.46 ± 0.38	<0.001 *
	Median	0.31	0.36	0.42 [†‡]	0.42	0.34	
Percentage (%)	Within ±0.25 D	47.1	38.6	24.3 [†]	27.1	40.0	0.015 *
	Within ±0.50 D	65.7	71.4	52.9	57.1	62.9	0.068
	Within ±1.00 D	95.7	92.9	92.9	88.6	90.0	0.28

* Significant difference among the formulas, calculated using Friedman test for the values and Cochran's Q test for the percentages. [†,‡,§,∥] Significant difference from Hill-RBF 3.0, Kane, BUII, and Haigis in post hoc analysis, respectively, calculated using pairwise Wilcoxon signed-rank test for the values and the McNemar test for the percentages with Bonferroni correction. BUII = Barrett Universal II; SD = standard deviation; D = diopters. Wang Koch adjustment was applied for the Haigis and SRK/T formulas.

Figure 1B shows the absolute error with each formula. The values with the Hill-RBF3.0 and Kane formula were smaller than that with the BUII formula, whereas there was not a statistically significant difference between the other formulas (Tables 2 and S1).

Figure 1C shows the stacked bar chart of the prediction accuracy with each formula. The percentage within ±0.25 D of the Hill-RBF3.0 formula was larger than that of the BUII (Tables 2 and S1).

Figure 2 shows the results of eyes with an AL > 28.0 mm. The prediction errors were significantly different from each other (Figure 2A, Tables 3 and S2). The absolute errors with the Hill-RBF3.0 and SRK/T were smaller than that with the Haigis formula (Figure 2B, Tables 3 and S2). The percentage within ±0.25 D with the Hill-RBF3.0 formula was larger than those with the Haigis formula (Figure 2C, Tables 3 and S2).

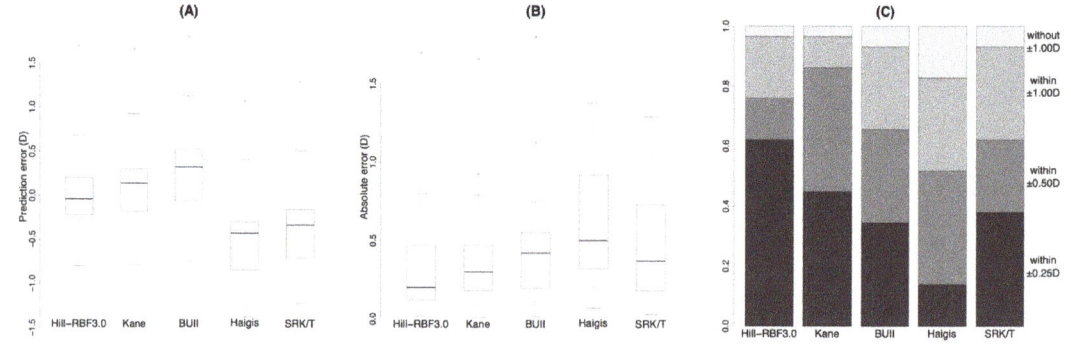

Figure 2. Prediction error (A), absolute error (B) and stacked bar chart (C) of prediction accuracy with each formula in eyes with axial length > 28.0 mm. BUII = Barrett Universal II; D = diopters. Wang Koch adjustment was applied for the Haigis and SRK/T formulas.

Table 3. Prediction accuracy with each formula in eyes with axial length > 28.0 mm.

		Hill-RBF3.0	Kane	BUII	Haigis	SRK/T	p-Value
Prediction error (D)	Mean ± SD	0.02 ± 0.48	0.10 ± 0.49	0.26 ± 0.50	−0.50 ± 0.50	−0.34 ± 0.49	<0.001 *
	Median	−0.04	0.14 [†]	0.32 [†,‡]	−0.43 [†,‡,§]	−0.34 [†,‡,§,∥]	
Absolute error (D)	Mean ± SD	0.33 ± 0.34	0.36 ± 0.34	0.43 ± 0.36	0.6 ± 0.36	0.48 ± 0.35	0.0015 *
	Median	0.20	0.30	0.42	0.50 [†]	0.37 [∥]	
Percentage (%)	Within ± 0.25 D	62.1	44.8	34.5	13.8 [†]	37.9	0.0029 *
	Within ± 0.50 D	75.9	86.2	65.5	51.7	62.1	0.012 *
	Within ± 1.00 D	96.6	96.6	93.1	82.8	93.1	0.044 *

* Significant difference between the formulas, calculated using Friedman test for the values and Cochran's Q test for the percentages. [†,‡,§,∥] Significant difference from Hill-RBF 3.0, Kane, BUII, and Haigis in post hoc analysis, respectively, calculated using pairwise Wilcoxon signed-rank test for the values and the McNemar test for the percentages with Bonferroni correction. BUII = Barrett Universal II; SD = standard deviation; D = diopters. Wang Koch adjustment was applied for the Haigis and SRK/T formulas.

Figure 3 shows a similar analysis in the subgroup of eyes with an AL < 28.0 mm. The median prediction errors with the Hill-RBF3.0 and Kane formulas were significantly different from those with other formulas, whereas there was not a statistically significant difference between those with the Hill-RBF3.0 and Kane formulas (Figure 3A, Tables 4 and S3). The absolute errors with the Hill-RBF3.0 and Kane formulas were smaller than that with the BUII formula (Figure 3B, Tables 4 and S3). The differences in the percentages among the formulas were not significantly different from each other (Figure 3C, Tables 4 and S3).

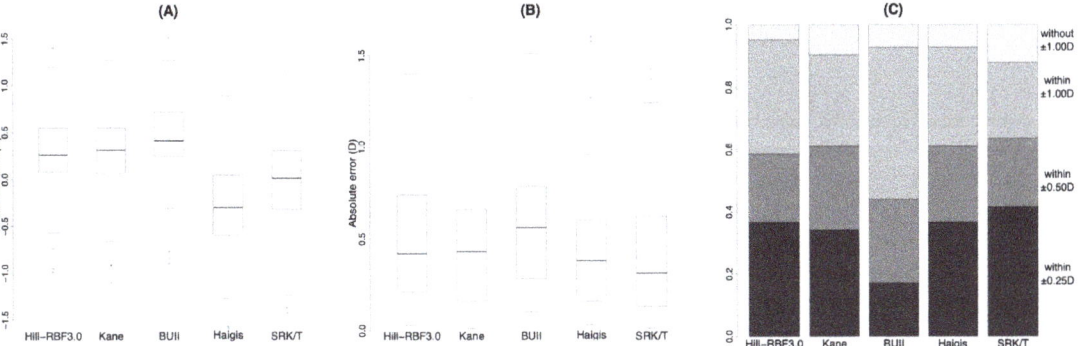

Figure 3. Prediction error (**A**), absolute error (**B**) and stacked bar chart (**C**) of prediction accuracy with each formula in eyes with axial length < 28.0 mm. BUII = Barrett Universal II; D = diopters. Wang Koch adjustment was applied for the Haigis and SRK/T formulas.

Table 4. Prediction accuracy with each formula in eyes with axial length < 28.0 mm.

		Hill-RBF3.0	Kane	BUII	Haigis	SRK/T	p-Value
Prediction error (D)	Mean ± SD	0.27 ± 0.53	0.25 ± 0.52	0.42 ± 0.50	−0.3 ± 0.52	−0.06 ± 0.61	<0.001 *
	Median	0.26	0.31	0.41 [†,‡]	−0.3 [†,‡,§]	0.01 [†,‡,§,∥]	
Absolute error (D)	Mean ± SD	0.49 ± 0.33	0.46 ± 0.34	0.57 ± 0.33	0.46 ± 0.38	0.45 ± 0.40	0.0017 *
	Median	0.42	0.43	0.56 [†,‡]	0.38	0.31	
Percentage (%)	Within ±0.25 D	36.6	34.1	17.1	36.6	41.5	0.12
	Within ±0.50 D	58.5	61.0	43.9	61.0	63.4	0.22
	Within ±1.00 D	95.1	90.2	92.7	92.7	87.8	0.60

* Significant difference between the formulas, calculated using Friedman test for the values and Cochran's Q test for the percentages. [†,‡,§,∥] Significant difference from Hill-RBF 3.0, Kane, BUII, and Haigis in post hoc analysis, respectively, calculated using pairwise Wilcoxon signed-rank test for the values and the McNemar test for the percentages with Bonferroni correction. BUII = Barrett Universal II; SD = standard deviation; D = diopters. Wang Koch adjustment was applied for the Haigis and SRK/T formulas.

4. Discussion

In the current study, the accuracy of the new formulas for IOL power calculations in highly myopic eyes (AL > 26.0 mm) was investigated in 70 uncomplicated cataract surgery cases. Overall, the prediction accuracy using AI (Hill-RBF3.0 and Kane) showed excellent prediction accuracy. Furthermore, this tendency was more obvious in eyes with an AL > 28.0 mm. No significant difference was observed in the prediction accuracy between the Hill-RBF3.0 and Kane formulas.

Theoretical formulas have been used for many years with continuous improvements. However, theoretical formulas are limited due to the measurement error of the AL or predicted postoperative anterior chamber depth (ACD), especially for eyes with long and short ALs outside the normal range. Recently, WK adjustment has been applied to myopic eyes [20]. The adjustment has been reported to reduce the amount of unexpected hyperopic surprise [2]. In the current study, SRK/T with WK adjustment showed excellent prediction accuracy, comparable to the new generation formulas.

Another possible approach to overcome this issue is by using AI, and the Hill-RBF and Kane formulas are representative of this approach. In the current study, these two formulas showed excellent prediction accuracy. Furthermore, this tendency was more obvious in long eyes with an AL > 28.0 mm. The Hill-RBF Calculator is a method for IOL power selection using pattern recognition and data interpolation. As more data are accumulated in the dataset, it is expected that the accuracy of this method will be further improved, and it will be able to calculate the powers for irregular cases. In fact, several negative studies have reported on the previous version of the Hill-RBF formula compared to the BUII formula [21,22]. However, in the current study, excellent prediction accuracy was observed with the updated formula. Even though there was no significant difference, only the Hill-RBF3.0 formula achieved prediction accuracy within ±0.25 D in more than half the cases in elongated eyes with an AL > 28.0 mm (Table 3). The biometric data used with the former version was AL, keratometry, and ACD, to which the central cornea thickness, lens thickness, white-to-white measurement and the sex of the patients could be added, although these were optional. These additional data were not used in the current study; however, the improved dataset with more parameters should improve the prediction accuracy of the model.

The current study has several limitations. We included a relatively small number of eyes. Although applying lens constant optimization was recommended [23], we did not do so in this study, since it was feasible only for four open-source formulas, i.e., the Haigis, Holladay 1, Hoffer Q, and SRK/T.

In conclusion, the prediction accuracy using AI (Hill-RBF3.0 and Kane) showed excellent prediction accuracy. No obvious difference was observed in the prediction accuracy between the Hill-RBF3.0 and Kane formulas.

5. Conclusions

This section is not mandatory but can be added to the manuscript if the discussion is unusually long or complex.

Supplementary Materials: The following supporting information can be downloaded at: https://www.mdpi.com/article/10.3390/jcm11164848/s1, Table S1: *p* Values in Post-Hoc Analyses. Table S2 *p*-Values in Post-Hoc Analyses in Eyes with Axial Length > 28.0 mm. Table S3: *p* Values in Post-Hoc Analyses in Eyes with Axial Length < 28.0 mm.

Author Contributions: Conceptualization, M.O., K.S., H.T., Y.N., E.Y. and K.N.; data curation, M.O., K.S., S.M., Y.S. and K.N.; Formal analysis, M.O.; Investigation, M.O. and K.N.; Methodology, M.O. and K.N.; project administration, K.N.; resources, K.S., H.T., S.M. and K.N.; supervision, K.S., H.T., S.M., Y.S., Y.N., E.Y. and K.N.; visualization, M.O.; writing—original draft, M.O.; writing—review and editing, K.S., H.T., S.M., Y.S., Y.N., E.Y. and K.N. All authors will be informed about each step of manuscript processing including submission, revision, revision reminder, etc., via emails from our system or assigned Assistant Editor. All authors have read and agreed to the published version of the manuscript.

Funding: This research received no external funding.

Institutional Review Board Statement: The study was conducted according to the guidelines of the Declaration of Helsinki and approved by the Institutional Review Board of Keio University (Protocol code; 20200141, date of approval; 29 July 2020).

Informed Consent Statement: All patients read and signed the written informed consent form at the institute before the surgery. Patient consent for participating in this study was waived and the opt-out approach was used according to the Ethical Guidelines for Medical and Health Research Involving Human Subjects presented by the Ministry of Education, Culture, Sports, Science and Technology in Japan.

Data Availability Statement: The data presented in this study are available on request from the corresponding author with the permission of the Keio University Ethics Committee. The data are stored, and will be discarded after the approved period by the Ethics Committee.

Conflicts of Interest: The authors declare no conflict of interest.

References

1. Haigis, W. Intraocular lens calculation in extreme myopia. *J. Cataract Refract. Surg.* **2009**, *35*, 906–911. [CrossRef] [PubMed]
2. Melles, R.B.; Holladay, J.T.; Chang, W.J. Accuracy of Intraocular Lens Calculation Formulas. *Ophthalmology* **2018**, *125*, 169–178. [CrossRef] [PubMed]
3. Dolgin, E. The myopia boom. *Nature* **2015**, *519*, 276–278. [CrossRef] [PubMed]
4. Morgan, I.G.; French, A.N.; Ashby, R.S.; Guo, X.; Ding, X.; He, M.; Rose, K.A. The epidemics of myopia: Aetiology and prevention. *Prog. Retin. Eye Res.* **2018**, *62*, 134–149. [CrossRef]
5. Morgan, I.G.; Ohno-Matsui, K.; Saw, S.-M. Myopia. *Lancet* **2012**, *379*, 1739–1748. [CrossRef]
6. Ji, J.; Liu, Y.; Zhang, J. Comparison of six methods for the intraocular lens power calculation in high myopic eyes. *Eur. J. Ophthalmol.* **2021**, *31*, 96–102. [CrossRef]
7. Liu, J.; Wang, L.; Chai, F.; Han, Y.; Qian, S.; Koch, D.D.; Weikert, M.P. Comparison of intraocular lens power calculation formulas in Chinese eyes with axial myopia. *J. Cataract Refract. Surg.* **2019**, *45*, 725–731. [CrossRef]
8. Omoto, M.K.; Torii, H.; Hayashi, K.; Ayaki, M.; Tsubota, K.; Negishi, K. Ratio of Axial Length to Corneal Radius in Japanese Patients and Accuracy of Intraocular Lens Power Calculation Based on Biometric Data. *Am. J. Ophthalmol.* **2020**, *218*, 320–329. [CrossRef]
9. Omoto, M.K.; Torii, H.; Masui, S.; Ayaki, M.; Tsubota, K.; Negishi, K. Ocular biometry and refractive outcomes using two swept-source optical coherence tomography-based biometers with segmental or equivalent refractive indices. *Sci. Rep.* **2019**, *9*, 6557. [CrossRef]
10. Wang, L.; Holladay, J.T.; Koch, D.D. Wang-Koch axial length adjustment for the Holladay 2 formula in long eyes. *J. Cataract Refract. Surg.* **2018**, *44*, 1291–1292. [CrossRef]
11. Wang, L.; Shirayama, M.; Ma, X.J.; Kohnen, T.; Koch, D.D. Optimizing intraocular lens power calculations in eyes with axial lengths above 25.0 mm. *J. Cataract Refract. Surg.* **2011**, *37*, 2018–2027. [CrossRef] [PubMed]
12. Warren, E.H. Hill-RBF Calculator Version 3.0. Available online: http://rbfcalculator.com/online/index.html (accessed on 1 May 2022).
13. Tsessler, M.; Cohen, S.; Wang, L.; Koch, D.D.; Zadok, D.; Abulafia, A. Evaluating the prediction accuracy of the Hill-RBF 3.0 formula using a heteroscedastic statistical method. *J. Cataract Refract. Surg.* **2021**, *48*, 37–43. [CrossRef] [PubMed]
14. Melles, R.B.; Kane, J.X.; Olsen, T.; Chang, W.J. Update on Intraocular Lens Calculation Formulas. *Ophthalmology* **2019**, *126*, 1334–1335. [CrossRef] [PubMed]
15. Bernardes, J.; Raimundo, M.; Lobo, C.; Murta, J.N. A Comparison of Intraocular Lens Power Calculation Formulas in High Myopia. *J. Refract Surg.* **2021**, *37*, 207–211. [CrossRef] [PubMed]
16. Cheng, H.; Wang, L.; Kane, J.X.; Li, J.; Liu, L.; Wu, M. Accuracy of Artificial Intelligence Formulas and Axial Length Adjustments for Highly Myopic Eyes. *Am. J. Ophthalmol.* **2021**, *223*, 100–107. [CrossRef] [PubMed]
17. Mo, E.; Lin, L.; Wang, J.; Huo, Q.; Yang, Q.; Liu, E.; Zhang, L.; Yu, Y.; Ye, L.; Pan, A.; et al. Clinical Accuracy of 6 Intraocular Lens Power Calculation Formulas in Elongated Eyes, According to Anterior Chamber Depth. *Am. J. Ophthalmol.* **2021**, *233*, 153–162. [CrossRef]
18. Popovic, M.; Schlenker, M.B.; Campos-Moller, X.; Pereira, A.; Ahmed, I.I.K. Wang-Koch formula for optimization of intraocular lens power calculation: Evaluation at a Canadian center. *J. Cataract Refract. Surg.* **2018**, *44*, 17–22. [CrossRef]
19. Wang, L.; Koch, D.D. Modified axial length adjustment formulas in long eyes. *J. Cataract Refract. Surg.* **2018**, *44*, 1396–1397. [CrossRef]
20. Kane, J.X.; Chang, D.F. Intraocular Lens Power Formulas, Biometry, and Intraoperative Aberrometry: A Review. *Ophthalmology* **2021**, *128*, e94–e114. [CrossRef]
21. Kane, J.X.; Van Heerden, A.; Atik, A.; Petsoglou, C. Accuracy of 3 new methods for intraocular lens power selection. *J. Cataract Refract. Surg.* **2017**, *43*, 333–339. [CrossRef]
22. Shajari, M.; Kolb, C.M.; Petermann, K.; Böhm, M.; Herzog, M.; de'Lorenzo, N.; Schönbrunn, S.; Kohnen, T. Comparison of 9 modern intraocular lens power calculation formulas for a quadrifocal intraocular lens. *J. Cataract Refract. Surg.* **2018**, *44*, 942–948. [CrossRef] [PubMed]
23. Hoffer, K.J.; Savini, G. Update on Intraocular Lens Power Calculation Study Protocols: The Better Way to Design and Report Clinical Trials. *Ophthalmology* **2021**, *128*, e115–e120. [CrossRef] [PubMed]

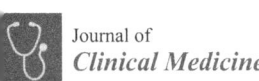

Journal of Clinical Medicine

Article

Evaluation of Visual and Patient—Reported Outcomes, Spectacle Dependence after Bilateral Implantation with a Non-Diffractive Extended Depth of Focus Intraocular Lens Compared to Other Intraocular Lenses

Anna Dołowiec-Kwapisz [1,*], Halina Piotrowska [1] and Marta Misiuk-Hojło [2]

[1] Department of Ophthalmology, Hospital in Zgorzelec, 59-900 Zgorzelec, Poland
[2] Department of Ophthalmology, Wrocław Medical University, 50-556 Wrocław, Poland
* Correspondence: annadolowiec@gmail.com

Abstract: Purpose: To evaluate postoperative outcomes, spectacle dependance and the occurrence of the photic phenomena in patients after cataract surgery following the implantation of a non-diffractive extended depth of focus (EDOF) intraocular lens was compared to monofocal and multifocal lenses. **Methods:** We enrolled patients with bilateral cataracts who wanted to reduce their dependence on glasses in the study. They were followed for 6 months. The study group in which the EDOF lens was implanted consisted of 70 eyes in 35 patients. The control groups consisted of: 52 eyes in 26 patients in whom a multifocal was implanted and 52 eyes in 26 patients with implanted monofocal lens. After a total of 2 weeks, 2 months and 6 months post-surgery the following were evaluated: uncorrected and corrected visual acuity at 4 m, 80 cm, 40 cm, manifest refraction expressed as mean refractive spherical equivalent (MRSE), contrast sensitivity, intraocular pressure. A questionnaire on independence from ocular correction, the occurrence of photic phenomena, and patient satisfaction was also completed. **Results**: Monocular and binocular visual acuity and MRSE 6 months after the procedure were compared between three groups. All of the main analyses, except for comparisons of uncorrected distance visual acuity (both monocular and binocular) level, were significant. Contrast sensitivity was lower among patients with multifocal lens than among patients with EDOF lens. Halo and glare after 6 months were seen more often among patients with multifocal lens than among patients with the other lens (65% of eyes with multifocal lens vs. 6% of eyes with EDOF lens and 0% of eyes with monofocal lens). Glasses were needed by 35% of patients with EDOF lens, and by 96% of patients with monofocal lens and in none of the patients with multifocal lens. **Conclusions**: Most patients qualify for the implantation of a non-diffractive EDOF lens. Post-operative visual acuity improves at any distance. The best monocular visual acuity for intermediate distances is provided by an EDOF lens, and for near distance by a multifocal lens. The EDOF lens definitely increases independence from spectacle correction compared to monofocal lenses; however, the greatest degree of independence from spectacles is provided by multifocal lenses. The incidence of photic phenomena is slightly higher than that of a monofocal lens, and much lower for a multifocal lens.

Keywords: cataract surgery; EDOF; intraocular lens; presbyopia; multifocal lens; photic phenomena

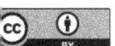

1. Introduction

Cataract surgery is one of the most frequently performed procedures around the world. Intraocular lenses (IOLs) have developed significantly in recent years. IOLs are used in cataract surgery to replace a cloudy lens and in refractive lens exchange (RLE). The most common implanted lenses are monofocal lenses, which provide good acuity to one type of vision correction, mainly for a far distance. In addition to monofocal lenses, premium lenses, which have a more advanced structure and different optical properties are available. These lenses correct presbyopia, i.e., insufficient accommodation that occurs physiologically after the age of 40. Premium lenses include multifocal intraocular lenses (MIOLs), extended depth of focus lenses (EDOF) and accommodative lenses. These lenses improve visual acuity after cataract surgery and allow for full or partial independence from spectacle correction. Both the extension of life expectancy, lifestyle changes and greater professional activity of the elderly contribute to the willingness to become independent from eyeglass correction not only in the distance, but also in the near and intermediate distance [1].

MIOLs allow for the greatest degree of independence from eyeglass correction, but they have a lower contrast sensitivity and a higher rate of photic phenomena, such as halo and glare. The eligibility criteria for implantation in this group of lenses are the most stringent, and the eyes should be free of any pathology so that patients can achieve the best possible postoperative results [2].

EDOF lenses can be positioned between monofocal and multifocal lenses. They provide good uncorrected distance and intermediate visual acuity; however, visual acuity without near correction may be insufficient. They work by creating a single, elongated focus to increase the depth of field. The elongated focus is designed to eliminate the close-up and distance overlap that occurs with multifocal lenses, thus eliminating the halo effect. In addition, EDOF lenses provide a continuous focus range, without the power distribution being unevenly divided, and thus avoiding secondary out-of-focus images [3,4]. Compared to multifocal lenses, they do not lower contrast sensitivity and cause less dysphotopsia [5].

There are different methods of creating these lenses. One of them is the use of spherical aberration, however, it differs from patient to patient in the population and is influenced by pupil width [6,7]. Another way is to use diffraction optics to obtain the EDOF effect. However, this can lead to the development of a dysfunction similar to those seen after multifocal lens implantation, and uncorrected near vision acuity may not be satisfactory [8]. Another method may be the use of a circular mask, as with the IC-8 lens, a small-aperture EDOF lens. However, this can reduce the amount of light entering through the diaphragm and is typically used in the non-dominant eye [9].

An increasing number of patients presenting for cataract surgery want to be independent from eyeglass correction, and at the same time are afraid of the photic phenomena after the procedure. There has been a growing number of patients after refractive surgery in the past who would like to regain independence from eyeglass correction and do not qualify for multifocal lens implantation. The same applies to patients with ocular diseases who would like to choose premium lenses. For these patients, EDOF lenses provide a chance to improve uncorrected acuity at all distances. Due to the fact that the EDOF Vivity lens (Alcon Laboratories, Inc., Fort Worth, TX, USA) has a unique, non-diffractive optical part; it allows patients to see well from near to distance. It is based on the non-diffractive X-wave technology, which modifies the wave front and creates one elongated focus without splitting the light. Thanks to these properties, the lens reduces the risk of dysphotopsia and does not worsen the contrast sensitivity. In the construction of the lens, two zones can be distinguished: the transition zone 1 is responsible for stretching the wave front and creating a continuous elongated focus, while the transition zone 2 is responsible for shifting the wave front from hyperopia to short-sighted in order to use all the light energy. It has 1.5 D defocusing and negative asphericity of the anterior surface (-0.2 μm) [10–12]. Moreover, the extended depth of focus, such as that seen in the Vivity lens, can "forgive" the imperfection of IOL power selection caused by the difficulty in calculating IOL power (especially in patients who have undergone refractive surgery in the past) [10].

To date, few articles have been published on postoperative outcomes in patients with non-diffractive EDOF lens implantation, including one in patients with ocular pathologies. This paper additionally includes patients with a history of refractive surgery, who will be increasingly more numerous in the future and would like to choose a premium lens. To the best of our knowledge, there are currently no publications on the comparison of the Vivity lens with monofocal and multifocal lenses. This work may provide some insight into lens selection, especially for patients with ocular pathologies and after refractive surgery who are ineligible for MIOLs or are worried about their side effects. The aim of the article is to evaluate the postoperative results, spectacle dependence, the occurrence of the photic phenomena in patients after cataract surgery using a non-diffractive EDOF–Vivity intraocular lens compared to multifocal and monofocal intraocular lenses.

2. Patients and Methods

2.1. Study Design

This single-center, prospective, comparative study was conducted at the Ophthalmology Department of the Hospital in Zgorzelec in line with the Helsinki Declaration and approved by the Bioethics Committee at the Medical University of Wroclaw. Written consent was obtained from all patients.

2.2. Study Population

The study group in which the Vivity lens was implanted (DFT015 or the toric version of the lens-called the EDOF group) consisted of 70 eyes in 35 patients. The control groups consisted of 52 eyes in 26 patients in whom a Panoptix multifocal lens (TNTF00 or the toric version of the lens-called the MULTI group) was implanted and 52 eyes in 26 patients with implanted monofocal lens (SA60WF or the toric version SN6AT3-7-called the MONO group). All lenses implanted in the patients involved in our study are single-piece, aspheric, are constructed of the same material-hydrophobic, and are based on the same platform-Acrysof (Alcon Laboratories, Inc., Fort Worth, TX, USA) [10,11,13–15]. The EDOF and multifocal lens were donated by the Alcon Company for the purpose of this study.

The study included patients aged 35–75 diagnosed with bilateral cataracts in whom the removal of the cataract was planned by phacoemulsification.

Exclusion criteria included: patients under the age of 35, over the age of 75, pregnant, after a corneal transplant, with a history of past eye injuries, diseases of the anterior and posterior segment of the eye that may have significantly reduced the quality of vision after surgery, such as: advanced glaucomatous neuropathy, advanced diabetic retinopathy, amblyopia, corneal scarring and dystrophy, exudative age-related macular degeneration (AMD), post-posterior vitrectomy condition or elective surgery, and clinically significant severe dry eye syndrome. Patients after cerebral events that could have affected visual acuity were also excluded from the study.

2.3. Preoperative Assessment

The pre-operative examination consisted of: anterior and posterior segment examination in a slit lamp, intraocular pressure examination, refraction examination (NIDEK ARK-510A-Nidek Co. Ltd., Gammagori, Aichi, Japan), monocular visual acuity examination in logarithm of the minimum angle of resolution (logMAR) scale: uncorrected distance visual acuity (UCDVA) at 4 m, best corrected distance visual acuity (BCDVA), uncorrected intermediate visual acuity (UCIVA) at 80 cm, best corrected intermediate visual acuity (BCIVA), uncorrected near visual acuity (UCNVA) with 40 cm, best corrected near visual acuity (BCNVA), monocular contrast sensitivity at 40 cm (Pelli-Robson test, GIMA charts, Gessate, Italy), biometry using an Argos SS-OCT optical biometer (Movu, Inc., Kamaki, Japan) and IOL Master 500 (Carl Zeiss Meditec AG, Jena, Germany), Oculazer™ WaveLight® II corneal tomography and topography (Alcon Laboratories, Inc., Fort Worth, TX, USA), posterior segment optical coherence tomography (OCT) (OCT III, Carl Zeiss Meditec AG, Jena, Germany). A standardized ETDRS chart at 4 m, 80 cm, and 40 cm was used to measure visual acuity (VA).

In the study, the refractive result was written as a spherical equivalent, defined as the sum of the spherical power and half of the cylindrical power [16]. The results obtained were classified as myopia, emmetropia or hyperopia. For myopia there was a spherical equivalent less than -0.5 D, for emmetropia-a spherical equivalent in the range of -0.5 and $+0.5$ D, and in the case of hyperopia, a spherical equivalent greater than $+0.5$ D. This division was adopted in accordance with other large cross-sectional and dynamic studies [16–18].

2.4. Postoperative Assessment

Controls were performed 2 weeks, 2 months (6–8 weeks) and 6 months after cataract surgery. Controls included: anterior and posterior segment examination in a slit lamp, an intraocular pressure test, manifest refraction expressed as mean refractive spherical equivalent (MRSE), monocular visual acuity test in the logMAR scale: UCDVA, BCDVA, UCIVA, BCIVA, UCNVA, BCNVA, monocular contrast sensitivity and the postoperative questionnaire.

Six months after the second eye surgery, binocular visual acuity was assessed: UCDVA, UCIVA, UCNVA.

Measurements were performed under photopic conditions (250–300 lumens/mm^2) in all cases. The preoperative and postoperative examinations were carried out by the same person.

2.5. Subjective Visual Quality Questionnaire

Patients were asked "yes/no" questions regarding independence from glasses, the occurrence of postoperative dysphotopsia such as halo, glare, starburst, was assesed on a scale from 1 to 5 in increments of 1 (1-slight, 5-very high). In addition, patients were asked to rate their satisfaction with the procedure (scale from 1 to 5).

2.6. Surgical Technique

All cataract surgery with implantation of an appropriate intraocular lens was performed by the same surgeon (H.P.). All the procedures were uneventful. They were performed under drip (Alcaine) and intraocular (Mydriane) anesthesia. The lenses were implanted through a 2.2 mm corneal incision into the lens bag. At the end of the procedure, in accordance with European standards, cefuroxime solution was administered into the anterior chamber.

Implant power for the Vivity lens was calculated on an Argos optical biometer using Barret's formula, setting postoperative results to either emmetropia (18 patients, 36 eyes) or minimonovision (17 patients, non-dominant eye set to target ~ −0.75D). Eye dominance was determined by taking the Mile's test. For Panoptix lenses, the Argos biometer and Barret's formula were used, setting postoperative results to emmetropia. Implant power of monofocal lenses was calculated using an IOL Master 500 or Argos biometer, using the SRK/T formula or the Barret formula by setting the target to emmetropia. With axial length <22 mm, the Haigis formula was used. In the case of patients after previous radial keratotomy, measurements were made on an Argos biometer using the Barret true K formula.

2.7. Statistical Analysis

All analyses were performed in statistical environment R, version 4.1.3. Quantitative variables were compared between groups with the Kruskal-Wallis test or with ANOVA analysis and between measurements—with the Friedman's test (for more than two measurements) or Wilcoxon's test for dependent samples (for two measurements). These tests were chosen because all variables' distributions significantly differed from the normal distribution (checked with Shapiro-Wilk's test). Median differences with 95% confidence intervals were given when comparing two measurements. Dependencies for qualitative variables were analyzed with the chi-square test or the Fisher's exact test. Significance level in the analysis equalled $\alpha = 0.05$.

3. Results

Pre- and postoperative data of 174 eyes (87 patients) were included in the analysis. A total of 35 patients (70 eyes) received the Vivity IOL (19 toric and 51 non-toric), 26 patients (52 eyes) underwent the implantation of monofocal (12 toric and 40 non-toric) lens, and 26 patients (52 eyes) the PanOptix lens (10 toric and 42 non-toric).

3.1. Demographics and Preoperative Data

Detailed demographic characteristics, biometry values, mean preoperative refractive errors and visual acuity (VA), contrast sensitivity, and intraocular pressure from the three groups are presented in Table 1.

Table 1. Demographics and preoperative characteristics (refractive and monocular VA (logMAR) data, ocular pathologies) of the three groups.

Variables	EDOF n = 70 Eyes n = 35 Subjects	MONO n = 52 Eyes n = 26 Subjects	MULTI n = 52 n = 26 Subjects	p	p^1	p^2	p^3
	Me (Q1; Q3) or M ± SD/n (%)						
Sex (female)	23 (65.7)	15 (57.7)	19 (73.1)	0.506	-	-	-
Age	57.74 ± 9.37	60.69 ± 10.65	59.46 ± 8.41	0.439 ^{2}	-	-	-
Refractive error							
Myopia	31 (44.3)	27 (51.9)	12 (23.1)	0.012 ^{1}	-	-	-
Emmetropia	5 (7.1)	2 (3.8)	9 (17.3)				
Hyperopia	34 (48.6)	23 (44.2)	31 (59.6)				
Axial lenght (mm)							
Short < 22	8 (11.4)	4 (7.7)	1 (1.9)	0.070 ^{1}	-	-	-
Medium 22–26	57 (81.4)	48 (92.3)	49 (94.2)				
Long > 26	5 (7.1)	0 (0.0)	2 (3.8)				
Toric IOL	19 (27.1)	12 (23.1)	10 (19.2)	0.606	-	-	-
MRSE (D)	0.50 (−2.50; 1.75)	−1.00 (−2.50; 2.31)	1.12 (−0.25; 2.00)	0.329	-	-	-
UCDVA	0.70 (0.30; 1.00)	0.70 (0.40; 0.77)	0.40 (0.29; 0.70)	**0.017**	0.624	**0.015**	**0.010**
BCDVA	0.25 (0.20; 0.30)	0.25 (0.25; 0.32)	0.25 (0.25; 0.25)	**0.004**	**0.005**	0.735	**0.002**
UCIVA	0.75 (0.43; 0.93)	0.60 (0.40; 0.90)	0.70 (0.48; 0.94)	0.236	-	-	-
BCIVA	0.20 (0.10; 0.40)	0.30 (0.10; 0.40)	0.20 (0.10; 0.30)	0.229	-	-	-
UCNVA	0.80 (0.70; 1.15)	0.70 (0.50; 0.86)	0.80 (0.60; 1.02)	0.054	-	-	-
BCNVA	0.30 (0.10; 0.50)	0.40 (0.20; 0.40)	0.20 (0.18; 0.32)	**0.014**	0.131	0.297	**0.001**
Contrast sensivity	1.80 (1.70; 1.90)	1.70 (1.58; 1.80)	1.80 (1.70; 1.83)	0.051	-	-	-
IOP (mmHg)	17.30 (16.25; 17.30)	17.30 (14.60; 17.30)	17.30 (14.60; 17.30)	0.270	-	-	-
ACD (mm)	3.15 (2.94; 3.52)	3.03 (2.80; 3.23)	3.17 (2.89; 3.36)	**0.012**	**0.003**	0.193	0.113
IOL power (D)	22.25 (19.50; 24.00)	23.00 (21.12; 23.62)	23.00 (21.00; 24.50)	0.553	-	-	-
Ocular pathology							
Glaucoma	4 (11.4)	8 (30.8)	2 (7.7)	0.0681	-	-	-
AMD	4 (11.4)	4 (15.4)	1 (3.8)	0.3751	-	-	-
Retinopathy	4 (11.4)	4 (15.4)	0 (0.0)	0.1171	-	-	-
Refractive surgery	4 (11.4)	0 (0.0)	0 (0.0)	0.0371	-	-	-

Table 1. Cont.

Variables	EDOF n = 70 Eyes n = 35 Subjects	MONO n = 52 Eyes n = 26 Subjects	MULTI n = 52 n = 26 Subjects	p	p^1	p^2	p^3
	Me (Q1; Q3) or M ± SD/n (%)						
PEX	2 (5.7)	2 (7.7)	4 (15.4)	0.5261	-	-	-
Drug-induced cataract	8 (22.9)	4 (15.4)	0 (0.0)	0.0251	-	-	-

Qualitative variables were described as n (%) and quantitative variables—as median with quartile 1 and 3 or mean with standard deviations. Dependencies between groups and qualitative variables were made using chi-square test or Fisher's exact test [1]. Comparisons of quantitative variables' level were made with Kruskal-Wallis test or with ANOVA [2] analysis. p—p value for main analyses; p value for post-hoc analyses: p^1—EDOF vs. MONO p^2—EDOF vs. MULTI, p^3—MONO vs. MULTI. Abbreviations: mm—milimiters, IOL—intraocular lens, AMD—age-related macular degeneration, PEX—pseudoexfoliation syndrome, MRSE—mean refraction spherical equivalent, D diopters, mmHg—millimetres of mercury, UCDVA—uncorrected distance visual acuity at 4 m, BCDVA—best corrected distance visual acuity, UCIVA—uncorrected intermediate visual acuity at 80 cm, BCIVA—best corrected intermediate visual acuity, UCNVA—uncorrected near visual acuity at 40 cm, BCNVA—best corrected near visual acuity.

Among the MULTI group there was a smaller proportion of eyes with myopia than in the other groups (23% vs. 44% for EDOF and 52% for MONO) and a higher proportion of eyes with emmetropia (17% vs. 7% for EDOF and 4% for MONO) or with hyperopia (60% vs. 49% for EDOF and 44% for MONO), p = 0.012. The analysis comparing quantitative variables was significant for: UCDVA (p = 0.017), BCDVA (p = 0.004), BCNVA (p = 0.014) and ACD (p = 0.012). Post-hoc analyses showed that patients from the MULTI group had a lower level of UCDVA variable than EDOF and MONO groups and lower level of BCNVA than the MONO group. Patients from the MONO group were characterized by a higher level of BCDVA than two remaining groups and by a lower level of ACD than patients from EDOF group (p < 0.050 for all post-hoc analyses), Table 1.

3.2. Refractive and Visual Outcomes

Monocular and binocular visual acuity and MRSE 6 months after the procedure were compared between EDOF, MONO and MULTI groups. All main analyses, except for comparisons of UCDVA (both monocular and binocular) level, were significant (p < 0.050). Post-hoc analyses showed that the level of: MRSE, BCDVA and BCIVA was higher among MULTI group than among EDOF group (p < 0.010 for all post-hoc analyses). Contrast sensitivity was lower among MULTI group than among EDOF group. The level of UCIVA (both monocular and binocular visual acuity) was higher in the MONO group than in the EDOF and MULTI groups (p < 0.001 for all post-hoc analyses) and higher in the MULTI group than in the EDOF group (p < 0.050 for both post-hoc analyses). The level of UCNVA (both monocular and binocular visual acuity) was higher in the MONO group than in the EDOF and MULTI groups (p < 0.001 for all post-hoc analyses) and higher in the EDOF group than in the MULTI group (p < 0.001 for both post-hoc analyses). The level of BCNVA was higher among MULTI group than among MONO group (p = 0.007), Table 2.

Table 2. Comparison of postoperative data (6 months after cataract surgery) between three groups.

Variables	EDOF	MONO	MULTI	p	p^1	p^2	p^3
	Me (Min–Max)						
MRSE (D)	−0.25 (−1.25; 0.50)	0.00 (−1.00; 0.75)	0.25 (−0.50; 0.75)	<0.001	0.053	<0.001	0.221
	Monocular visual acuity (logMAR)						
UCDVA	0.00 (−0.20; 0.20)	0.00 (−0.10; 0.40)	0.00 (−0.15; 0.20)	0.433	-	-	-

Table 2. Cont.

Variables	EDOF	MONO	MULTI	p	p^1	p^2	p^3
	Me (Min–Max)						
BCDVA	0.00 (−0.20; 0.00)	0.00 (−0.20; 0.00)	0.00 (−0.15; 0.00)	0.008	0.335	0.009	0.233
UCIVA	0.00 (−0.10; 0.30)	0.30 (−0.10; 0.60)	0.10 (−0.20; 0.30)	<0.001	<0.001	0.004	<0.001
BCIVA	0.00 (−0.10; 0.10)	0.00 (−0.20; 0.20)	0.00 (−0.20; 0.20)	0.008	0.590	0.004	0.331
UCNVA	0.40 (0.00; 0.60)	0.50 (0.10; 0.90)	0.10 (0.00; 0.20)	<0.001	<0.001	<0.001	<0.001
BCNVA	0.00 (−0.10; 0.20)	0.00 (−0.10; 0.10)	0.00 (0.00; 0.30)	0.008	0.301	0.229	0.007
	Binocular visual acuity (logMAR)						
UCDVA	0.00 (−0.15; 0.10)	0.00 (−0.10; 0.14)	0.00 (−0.15; 0.10)	0.767	-	-	-
UCIVA	0.00 (−0.10; 0.10)	0.20 (−0.20; 0.40)	0.00 (−0.10; 0.14)	<0.001	<0.001	0.015	<0.001
UCNVA	0.26 (0.00; 0.46)	0.40 (0.04; 0.70)	0.00 (0.00; 0.10)	<0.001	<0.001	<0.001	<0.001
Contrast sensitivity	2.00 (1.80; 2.00)	2.00 (1.80; 2.00)	1.90 (1.80; 2.00)	<0.001	0.907	<0.001	0.063

Variables were described as median with range of scores (min–max). Comparisons of quantitative variables' level were made with Kruskal-Wallis test. p—p value for main analyses; p value for post-hoc analyses: p^1—EDOF vs. MONO, p^2—EDOF vs. MULTI, p^3—MONO vs. MULTI.

When the EDOF group is divided into two subgroups: (1) patients with target set to emmetropia, (2) patients with minimonovision (non-dominant eye set to target ca. −0.75 D) the results of binocular uncorrected visual acuity 6 months after surgery are as follows, Table 3.

Table 3. Comparison of uncorrected binocular acuity at all distances between four groups (EDOF group divided into 2 subgroups: emmetropia i minimonovision).

Variables	Emmetropia	Minimonovision	MONO	MULTI	p for Main Analyses
	Me (Q1; Q3)				
UCDVA	0.00 (−0.09; 0.00)	0.00 (−0.10; 0.00)	0.00 (−0.06; 0.00)	0.00 (−0.09; 0.00)	0.904
UCIVA	0.00 (0.00; 0.03)	0.00 (−0.06; 0.00)	0.20 (0.10; 0.24)	0.00 (0.00; 0.06)	<0.001
UCNVA	0.30 (0.22; 0.36)	0.20 (0.10; 0.30)	0.40 (0.30; 0.50)	0.00 (0.00; 0.03)	<0.001
	p value for post-hoc analyses				
				UCIVA	UCNVA
Emmetropia vs. minimonovision				0.040	0.062
Emmetropia vs. MONO				<0.001	0.001
Emmetropia vs. MULTI				0.172	<0.001
Minimonovision vs. MONO				<0.001	<0.001
Minimonovision vs. MULTI				<0.001	<0.001
MONO vs. MULTI				<0.001	<0.001

Variables were described as median with quartile 1 and 3. Comparisons of quantitative variables' level were made with Kruskal-Wallis test.

Refractive and Visual Outcomes in Baseline and after 6 Months in Each Group

In the EDOF group at the baseline the level of: UCDVA (MD 95% CI = 0.70 (0.63; 0.82); $p < 0.001$), BCDVA (MD 95% CI = 0.25 (0.30; 0.35); $p < 0.001$), UCIVA (MD 95% CI = 0.75 (0.64; 0.80); $p < 0.001$), BCIVA (MD 95% CI = 0.20 (0.25; 0.35); $p < 0.001$), UCNVA (MD 95% CI = 0.40 (0.45; 0.60); $p < 0.001$), BCNVA (MD 95% CI = 0.30 (0.25; 0.40); $p < 0.001$) and IOP (MD 95% CI − 2.85 (1.90; 3.00); $p < 0.001$) was higher than after 6 months. The level of contrast was lower at the baseline than after 6 months (MD 95% CI = −0.20 (−0.35; −0.20); $p < 0.001$).

In the MONO group almost all comparisons between baseline and after 6 months were significant (except of the MRSE level). At the baseline the level of: UCDVA (MD 95% CI = 0.70 (0.55; 0.75); $p < 0.001$), BCDVA (MD 95% CI = 0.25 (0.30; 0.38); $p < 0.001$), UCIVA (MD 95% CI = 0.30 (0.30; 0.50); $p < 0.001$), BCIVA (MD 95% CI = 0.30 (0.24; 0.33); $p < 0.001$), UCNVA (MD 95% CI = 0.20 (0.13; 0.33); $p < 0.001$), BCNVA (MD 95% CI = 0.40 (0.30; 0.40); $p < 0.001$) and IOP (MD 95% CI = 2.80 (0.85; 2.45); $p < 0.001$) was higher than after 6 months. The level of contrast sensitivity was lower at the baseline than after 6 months (MD 95% CI = −0.30 (−0.35; −0.25); $p < 0.001$).

All analyses were significant in the case of the MULTI group. At the baseline the level of: MRSE (MD 95% CI = 0.87 (0.00; 1.37); $p = 0.043$), UCDVA (MD 95% CI = 0.40 (0.40; 0.57); $p < 0.001$), BCDVA (MD 95% CI = 0.25 (0.25; 0.28); $p < 0.001$), UCIVA (MD 95% CI = 0.60 (0.60; 0.80); $p < 0.001$), BCIVA (MD 95% CI = 0.20 (0.15; 0.25); $p < 0.001$), UCNVA (MD 95% CI = 0.70 (0.65; 0.80); $p < 0.001$), BCNVA (MD 95% CI = 0.20 (0.20; 0.25); $p < 0.001$) and IOP (MD 95% CI = 2.90 (1.55; 2.50); $p < 0.001$) was higher than after 6 months. The level of contrast sensitivity was again lower at the baseline than after 6 months (MD 95% CI = −0.10 (−0.20; −0.15); $p < 0.001$)

3.3. Evaluation of Dysphotopsia

Halo and glare after 6 months were experienced more often among subjects form the MULTI group than among subjects from the two other groups (65% of eyes in MULTI group vs. 6% of eyes in the EDOF group and 0% of eyes in the MONO group; $p < 0.001$ for halo and 10% of eyes in the MULTI group vs. 3% of eyes in the EDOF group and 0% of eyes in the MONO group; $p = 0.045$). No other significant difference was detected between groups and between the occurrence of photic phenomena 6 months after the procedure, Table 4.

Table 4. Comparison of occurrence of photic phenomena 6 months after the procedure between three groups.

Variables	EDOF n = 70 Eyes	MONO n = 52 Eyes	MULTI n = 52 Eyes	p
		n (%)		
Halo	4 (5.7)	0 (0.0)	34 (65.4)	<0.001 [2]
Halo level				
1	1 (25.0)	-	13 (38.2)	
2	3 (75.0)	-	12 (35.3)	
3	0 (0.0)	-	8 (23.5)	0.563
4	0 (0.0)	-	1 (2.9)	
5	0 (0.0)	-	0 (0.0)	
Glare	2 (2.9)	0 (0.0)	5 (9.6)	0.045
Glare level				
1	0 (0.0)	-	4 (80.0)	
2	1 (50.0)	-	1 (20.0)	
3	1 (50.0)	-	0 (0.0)	0.143
4	0 (0.0)	-	0 (0.0)	
5	0 (0.0)	-	0 (0.0)	
Starburst	4 (5.7)	2 (3.8)	8 (15.4)	0.097
Starburst level				
1	1 (25.0)	0 (0.0)	2 (25.0)	
2	3 (75.0)	2 (100.0)	4 (50.0)	
3	0 (0.0)	0 (0.0)	2 (25.0)	0.899
4	0 (0.0)	0 (0.0)	0 (0.0)	
5	0 (0.0)	0 (0.0)	0 (0.0)	

Variables were described as n (%). Dependencies between groups and qualitative variables were made using chi-square test [2] or Fisher's exact test.

3.4. Spectacle Dependence and Patient Satisfaction

Glasses were needed by 35% of subjects from the EDOF group, by 96% of subjects from the MONO group and by no one from the MULTI group (this was a statistically significant dependency—$p < 0.001$). Every patient from every group was satisfied (both for the right and left the eye). Most of subjects from each group rated their satisfaction (both for right and left eye) with a number 5 (97% for right eye and 86% for left eye in the EDOF group; 92% for right eye and 81% for left eye in the MONO group; 77% for right eye and 85% for left eye in the MULTI group; $p = 0.552$ for the dependency between groups and level of satisfaction for right eye and $p > 0.999$ for the dependency between groups and level of satisfaction for left eye). Among the MULTI group, there was a greater proportion of subjects that rated their satisfaction for the right eye with the number 4 than in two other groups (23% vs. 3% in EDOF and 8% in MONO; $p = 0.038$), Table 5.

Table 5. Number of patients needing glasses and satisfaction rating broken down by groups.

Variable	EDOF n = 35 Subjects	MONO n = 26 Subjects	MULTI n = 26 Subjects	p
		n (%)		
Glasses	14 (35.0)	25 (96.2)	0 (0.0)	<0.001 [2]
Satisfaction (right eye)	35 (100.0)	26 (100.0)	26 (100.0)	-
Satisfaction (left eye)	35 (100.0)	26 (100.0)	26 (100.0)	-
Level of satisfaction (right eye)				
1	0 (0.0)	0 (0.0)	0 (0.0)	
2	0 (0.0)	0 (0.0)	0 (0.0)	
3	0 (0.0)	0 (0.0)	0 (0.0)	0.038
4	1 (2.9)	2 (7.7)	6 (23.1)	
5	34 (97.1)	24 (92.3)	20 (76.9)	
Level of satisfaction (left eye)				
1	0 (0.0)	0 (0.0)	0 (0.0)	
2	0 (0.0)	0 (0.0)	0 (0.0)	
3	0 (0.0)	0 (0.0)	0 (0.0)	0.932
4	5 (14.3)	5 (19.2)	4 (15.4)	
5	30 (85.7)	21 (80.8)	22 (84.6)	

Dependencies were calculated using chi-square test [2] or Fisher's exact test.

4. Discussion

4.1. Qualification

Due to the non-diffractive structure of the lens and one elongated focus, the EDOF lens can be implanted in patients who do not qualify for multifocal lens implantation or are afraid of either the photic phenomena or reduced contrast sensitivity. In the case of multifocal lenses, the eligibility criteria are the strictest, and patients should be free of ocular diseases in order to achieve the best possible vision after surgery. As can be seen in Table 1, the patients who were qualified for cataract surgery with a non-diffractive EDOF lens had eyes with various ocular pathologies or past refractive surgeries, which did not impair the prognosis for improved vision after surgery, and thus patient satisfaction after surgery was high. The profile of patients in this case is similar to that of patients qualified for surgery with monofocal lens implantation.

4.2. Postoperative Results

The non-diffractive EDOF lens provides good acuity of distance vision, intermediate distance and functional near vision, confirmed by previous studies [19]. In our study, patients who had the Vivity lens implanted achieved a significant improvement in VA at all distances. The UCDVA at 4 m monocular is similar between the EDOF, the MONO group and the MULTI group. In the case of the monocular UCIVA at 80 cm, VA is better for patients in the EDOF group than for the MONO and MULTI groups (UCIVA EDOF = 0.0, MULTI = 0.1, MONO = 0.3, respectively). In the case of monocular UCNVA, patients in the EDOF group achieved a worse VA than patients in the MULTI group and better than in the MONO group, as confirmed by other published studies comparing EDOF lenses with multifocal and monofocal lenses [15,19–21]. The worse monocular UCIVA at 80 cm for the MULTI group compared to the EDOF group may be due to the fact that the PanOptix lens has a focus to intermediate distance at 60 cm [15].

To the best of our knowledge, no study has been published, comparing at the same time the Vivity lens with monofocal and multifocal to date. In a large randomized study, Bal C. et al. compared postoperative outcomes in patients implanted with a Vivity lens compared to an aspheric monofocal lens. They described better intermediate and near distance vision after implantation of the Vivity lens and a similar visual impairment profile compared to the aspheric monofocal IOL [20].

In the study by Kohnen T. et al. the postoperative outcomes after bilateral Vivity lens implantation with target refraction set to emmetropia were assessed (32 eyes—16 patients). Patients achieved: binocular uncorrected VA for distance, intermediate distance and near distance, respectively, 0.01 ± 0.05 logMAR at 4 m, 0.05 ± 0.05 logMAR at 80 cm, 0.07 ± 0.06 logMAR at 66 cm and 0.25 ± 0.11 logMAR at 40 cm [22]. The results obtained in our study, for EDOF lens implantation with target refraction set to emmetropia were very similar (Me [Q1; Q3]): binocular UDCVA at 4 m 0.00 (−0.09; 0.00) logMAR, binocular UCIVA at 80 cm 0.00 (0.00; 0.03) logMAR, and binocular UCNVA at 40 cm 0.30 (0.22; 0.36) logMAR, respectively.

Arrigo A. et al. describes the authors' own experiences in healthy eyes (108 eyes—54 patients) after EDOF Vivity lens implantation. Very good results of distance vision and intermediate distance were described; in the case of near vision, the need for an addition of at least +1.0 D was indicated. Monocular UCDVA was 0.1 ± 0.04 logMAR, monocular BCDVA was 0.0 ± 0.03 logMAR, respectively [23]. Patients in our study with an implanted Vivity lens also needed a near vision supplement of about 1D or more and median monocular UCDVA was 0.0 logMAR, median monocular BCDVA was 0.0 logMAR.

The use of the minimonovision system in the case of the Vivity lens improves the VA for near vision and increases the degree of independence from ocular correction. In the paper by Newsom T. et al. describing the results of binocular Vivity lens implantation with target of slight myopia −0.75 D, 29 of 33 eyes achieved UCNVA binocular 0.2 logMAR or better [24]. Very similar results were obtained in our patients wih minimovision, whose median binocular UCNVA was 0.2 logMAR.

Rementería-Capelo LA et al. describes the postoperative results after binocular Vivity lens implantation in patients with ocular pathology. A monocular UCDVA was achieved in the test group of 0.03 ± 0.8 logMAR, compared to the control group with an implanted Vivity lens without eye pathology -0.1 ± 0.07. The statistical difference between binocular UCDVA in both groups was not described, as was the case of defocus curves and contrast sensitivity [25]. The result of this study is similar to ours, which evaluated the visual acuity of both healthy patients and those with ocular pathology (median of monocular and binocular UCDVA was 0.0 logMAR). These results, although described on small groups and with a wide range of ocular disorders, give evidence that ocular disorders do not disqualify from Vivity lens implantation. Postoperative results in these patients are very good.

4.3. Spectacle Dependance

Therefore, EDOF lenses can be positioned between monofocal and multifocal lenses they provide good uncorrected visual acuity for distance and intermediate, but uncorrected visual acuity for nearsightedness may be insufficient. In our study, glasses were needed by 35% of subjects from the EDOF group, by 96% of subjects from the MONO group and by no one from the MULTI group (this was a statistically significant dependency—$p < 0.001$) In a study by Rementería-Capelo LA et al., 40% of patients in both study groups (with and without ocular pathology) reported never using close-up glasses [25]. Similar results were described by Kohnen et al. (38%) [22]. The higher degree of independence from spectacle correction among our patients with EDOF lens implantation may be due to the different profile of qualified patients for the procedure. In addition, our EDOF group was not a homogeneous group and some patients had the target set to emmetropia and some had the minimovision system applied. This was due to patient preference and their desire to improve their near vision. In addition, each patient prefers a different reading distance, which also contributes to the different results.

As you know, the use of a minimovision system in the cases of the Vivity lens improves near vision acuity and increases the degree of independence from spectacle correction. Newsom T. et described a high level of satisfaction and a greater degree of independence from ocular correction with the monovision system than without monovision with implantation of the same lens [24].

4.4. Occurance of Photic Phenomena

In our study, a small number of patients after EDOF implantation reported photic phenomena (14% patients). Patients who reported the occurrence of dysphotopsia described these side effects as minor, not disrupting normal functioning, similar to the previous reports [20,22,23]. Compared to patients in the MONO group, the incidence of dysphotopsia is slightly more frequent, but it is definitely seen less than in patients in the MULTI group. The study by Rementería-Capelo LA et al. described that patients reported a higher prevalence of halos and glare than other reports on Vivity IOL, especially in the study group, with ocular pathologies: 60% halo, 54% glare, compared to the control group, where the incidence of halo was 28% and 48% [25]. Kohnen et al. found that 25% reported halo and 25% glare [22]. Arrigo et al. reported that 30% and 33% of patients reported halo and glare [23]. The differences between the studies may be due to differences in the questionnaires used in the study and the "inquiry," an active question about the presence of dysphotopsia, and this has been shown to increase reporting rates [26].

A paper by Newsom T. et described that the use of a monovision system when implanting a Vivity lens compared to target refraction set to emmetropia does not increase the frequency of photic phenomena [24].

4.5. Contrast Sensivity

Although this was not the main aim in the study also described was the contrast sensivity. Some patients, due to the fear of decreased of contrast sensivity after surgery, choose not to implant multifocal lenses and select EDOF lenses. According to the manufacturer, the Vivity lens has a safety profile similar to that of monofocal lenses [11,19]. In our study, contrast sensitivity in patients implanted with the Vivity lens did not differ significantly from patients implanted with a monofocal lens and was better than that of patients implanted with a multifocal lens. It is difficult to relate the results of this study to others, since contrast sensitivity was tested only with nearsighted charts and only under photopic conditions.

In our study, we encountered a few limitations. First, it was conducted at a single center, so the number of patients in the study was limited. Secondly, each study group included both healthy patients and patients with eye pathology and after refractive surgery. Studies focusing on specific ocular pathologies or on patients after specific refractive procedures, with larger numbers of patients, would be necessary to best determine which type of IOL would provide the greatest benefit for a given group of patients. In addition, comparing data from our study with other published studies is problematic due to different inclusion/exclusion criteria, study conditions and procedures.

5. Conclusions

The majority of patients presenting for cataract surgery who wished to increase independence from spectacle correction are eligible for the implantation of a non-diffractive

EDOF lens. Postoperative visual acuity improves at any distance. In the case of the monocular uncorrected intermediate visual acuity at 80 cm, it is better for patients with EDOF lens than with monocofal or multifocal lens. In the case of monocular uncorrected near visual acuity at 40 cm, patients with EDOF lens achieved worse visual acuity than patients with multifocal lens and better than with monofocal lens. The EDOF lens definitely increases independence from spectacle correction compared to monofocal lenses (65% vs 4%); however, the greatest degree of independence from spectacles is provided by multifocal lenses (100%). Only 14% patients after EDOF implantation reported photic phenomena. Compared to patients with monofocal lens, the incidence of dysphotopsia is slightly more frequent, but definitely it is seen less than in patients with multifocal lens.

Author Contributions: Conceptualization, A.D.-K.; methodology: A.D.-K., H.P., M.M.-H.; investigation, A.D.-K. and H.P.; data curation, A.D.-K.; writing—original draft preparation, A.D.-K.; writing—review and editing, H.P. and M.M.-H.; supervision M.M.-H. All authors have read and agreed to the published version of the manuscript.

Funding: The APC was funded by NS Marketing Anna Malecka, Olesińska street 21/116, 02-548 Warszawa, NIP 971-048-44-6.

Institutional Review Board Statement: The study was conducted in accordance with the Declaration of Helsinki, and approved by the Bioethics Committee at the Medical University of Wroclaw, 759/2021, approval date: 17 September 2021.

Informed Consent Statement: Informed consent was obtained from all subjects involved in the study.

Data Availability Statement: Not applicable.

Acknowledgments: The authors would like to thank the patients for providing written informed consent to publish this article and for the contribution of valuable supporting information from his medical records.

Conflicts of Interest: The authors declare no conflict of interest.

References

1. Misiuk-Hojło, M.; Dołowiec-Kwapisz, A. Patient with Cataract—Observations after 2 Years of the Pandemic and Future Prospects. Ophthatherapy. 11 May 2022. Available online: https://www.journalsmededu.pl/index.php/ophthatherapy/article/view/1793 (accessed on 30 May 2022).
2. Alió, J.L.; Plaza-Puche, A.B.; Férnandez-Buenaga, R.; Pikkel, J.; Maldonado, M. Multifocal intraocular lenses: An overview. *Surv. Ophthalmol.* **2017**, *62*, 611–634. [CrossRef] [PubMed]
3. Savini, G.; Balducci, N.; Carbonara, C.; Rossi, S.; Altieri, M.; Frugis, N.; Zappulla, E.; Bellucci, R.; Alessio, G. Functional assessment of a new extended depth-of-focus intraocular lens. *Eye* **2019**, *33*, 404–410. [CrossRef]
4. Savini, G.; Schiano-Lomoriello, D.; Balducci, N.; Barboni, P. Visual performance of a new extended depth-of-focus intraocular lens compared to a distance-dominant diffractive multifocal intraocular lens. *J. Refract. Surg.* **2018**, *34*, 228–235. [CrossRef] [PubMed]
5. Kohnen, T.; Suryakumar, R. Extended depth-of-focus technology in intraocular lenses. *J. Cataract Refract. Surg.* **2020**, *46*, 298–304. [CrossRef] [PubMed]
6. Bellucci, R.; Cargnoni, M.; Bellucci, C. Clinical and aberrometric evaluation of a new extended depth-of-focus intraocular lens based on spherical aberration. *J. Cataract Refract. Surg.* **2019**, *45*, 919–926. [CrossRef] [PubMed]
7. Fernández, J.; Rodríguez-Vallejo, M.; Burguera, N.; Rocha-de-lossada, C.; Piñero, D.P. Spherical aberration for expanding depth of focus. *J. Cataract Refract. Surg.* **2021**, *47*, 1587–1595. [CrossRef] [PubMed]
8. Singh, B.; Sharma, S.; Dadia, S.; Bharti, N.; Bharti, S. Comparative evaluation of visual outcomes after bilateral implantation of a diffractive trifocal intraocular lens and an extended depth of focus intraocular lens. *Eye Contact Lens* **2020**, *46*, 314–318. [CrossRef] [PubMed]
9. Hooshmand, J.; Allen, P.; Huynh, T.; Chan, C.; Singh, R.; Moshegov, C.; Agarwal, S.; Thornell, E.; Vote, B.J. Small aperture IC-8 intraocular lens in cataract patients: Achieving extended depth of focus through small aperture optics. *Eye* **2019**, *33*, 1096–1103. [CrossRef] [PubMed]
10. Dołowiec-Kwapisz, A.; Misiuk-Hojło, M.; Piotrowska, H. Cataract Surgery after Radial Keratotomy with Non-Diffractive Extended Depth of Focus Lens Implantation. *Medicina* **2022**, *58*, 689. [CrossRef]
11. Alcon Data on File, 2019–2020; AcrySof® IQ Vivity™ Extended Vision IOL Directions for Use. Alcon Laboratories, Inc. 2020. Available online: https://www.accessdata.fda.gov/cdrh_docs/pdf/p970003.pdf (accessed on 28 May 2022).
12. Gundersen, K.G.; Potvin, R. Clinical Outcomes and Quality of Vision Associated with Bilateral Implantation of a Wavefront Shaping Presbyopia Correcting Intraocular Lens. *Clin. Ophthalmol.* **2021**, *15*, 4723–4730. [CrossRef]

3. Alcon Laboratories, Inc. *Product Information: AcrySof Aspheric UV-Absorbing Single-Piece IOL: SA60WF*; Alcon Laboratories, Inc.: Geneva, Switzerland. Available online: http://embed.widencdn.net/pdf/plus/alcon/vmjmutqbkm/40-500-214_us_en.pdf?u=4rqn9d (accessed on 30 May 2022).
4. Alcon Laboratories, Inc. *Product Information: Acrysof IQ Toric, Astigmatism IOL, STERILE UV and Blue Light Filtering Acrylic Foldable Toric Aspheric Optic Single-Piece Posterior Chamber Lenses*; Alcon Laboratories, Inc.: Geneva, Switzerland. Available online: http://embed.widencdn.net/pdf/plus/alcon/apcard9uoq/40-500-143_us_en.pdf?u=4rqn9d (accessed on 30 May 2022).
5. Sudhir, R.R.; Dey, A.; Bhattacharrya, S.; Bahulayan, A. AcrySof IQ PanOptix Intraocular Lens Versus Extended Depth of Focus Intraocular Lens and Trifocal Intraocular Lens: A Clinical Overview. *Asia-Pac. J. Ophthalmol.* **2019**, *8*, 335–349. [CrossRef]
6. Guzowski, M.; Wang, J.J.; Rochtchina, E.; Rose, K.A.; Mitchell, P. Five-year refractive changes in an older population. *Ophthalmology* **2003**, *110*, 1364–1370. [CrossRef]
7. Attebo, K.; Ivers, R.Q.; Mitchell, P. Refractive errors in an older population. *Ophthalmology* **1999**, *106*, 1066–1072. [CrossRef]
8. Gürbüz Yurtseven, Ö.; Aksoy, S.; Karatay Arsan, A.; Buyru Özkurt, Y.; Kökçen, H.K. Evaluation of the Relationship Between Age-related Macular Degeneration and Refractive Error, Socio-demographic Features, and Biochemical Variables in a Turkish Population. *Turk. J. Ophthalmol.* **2018**, *48*, 238–244. [CrossRef]
9. US FDA. AcrySof™ IQ Vivity™ Extended Vision Intraocular Lens (IOL): Summary of Safety and Effectiveness Data. Available online: https://www.accessdata.fda.gov/cdrh_docs/pdf/P930014S126B.pdf (accessed on 30 May 2022).
10. Bala, C.; Poyales, F.; Guarro, M.; Mesa, R.R.; Mearza, A.; Varma, D.K.; Jasti, S.; Lemp-Hull, J. Multicountry clinical outcomes of a new nondiffractive presbyopia-correcting IOL. *J. Cataract Refract. Surg.* **2022**, *48*, 136–143. [CrossRef]
11. Sieburth, R.; Chen, M. Intraocular lens correction of presbyopia. *Taiwan J. Ophthalmol.* **2019**, *9*, 4–17. [CrossRef] [PubMed]
12. Kohnen, T.; Petermann, K.; Böhm, M.; Hemkeppler, E.; Ahmad, W.; Hinzelmann, L.; Pawlowicz, K.; Jandewerth, T.; Lwowski, C. Nondiffractive wavefront-shaping extended depth-of-focus intraocular lens: Visual performance and patient-reported outcomes. *J. Cataract Refract. Surg.* **2022**, *48*, 144–150. [CrossRef] [PubMed]
13. Arrigo, A.; Gambaro, G.; Fasce, F.; Aragona, E.; Figini, I.; Bandello, F. Extended depth-of-focus (EDOF) AcrySof® IQ Vivity® intraocular lens implant: A real-life experience. *Graefes Arch. Clin. Exp. Ophthalmol.* **2021**, *259*, 2717–2722. [CrossRef]
14. Newsom, T.H.; Potvin, R. Evaluation of Quality of Vision and Visual Outcomes with Bilateral Implantation of a Non-Diffractive Extended Vision Intraocular Lens with a Target of Slight Myopia in the Non-Dominant Eye. *Clin. Ophthalmol.* **2022**, *16*, 183–190. [CrossRef]
15. Rementería-Capelo, L.A.; Lorente, P.; Carrillo, V.; Sánchez-Pina, J.M.; Ruiz-Alcocer, J.; Contreras, I. Patient Satisfaction and Visual Performance in Patients with Ocular Pathology after Bilateral Implantation of a New Extended Depth of Focus Intraocular Lens. *J. Ophthalmol.* **2022**, *2022*, 4659309. [CrossRef]
16. Makhotkina, N.Y.; Nijkamp, M.D.; Berendschot, T.T.J.M.; van den Borne, B.; Nuijts, R.M.M.A. Effect of active evaluation on the detection of negative dysphotopsia after sequential cataract surgery: Discrepancy between incidences of unsolicited and solicited complaints. *Acta Ophthalmol.* **2018**, *96*, 81–87. [CrossRef] [PubMed]

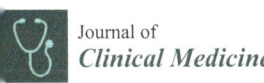

Article

Accuracy of Six Intraocular Lens Power Calculations in Eyes with Axial Lengths Greater than 28.0 mm

Majid Moshirfar [1,2,3,*], Kathryn M. Durnford [4], Jenna L. Jensen [4], Daniel P. Beesley [5], Telyn S. Peterson [6], Ines M. Darquea [1], Yasmyne C. Ronquillo [1] and Phillip C. Hoopes [1]

1. Hoopes Vision, HDR Research Center, Draper, UT 84020, USA
2. John A. Moran Eye Center, Department of Ophthalmology and Visual Sciences, Salt Lake City, UT 84132, USA
3. Utah Lions Eye Bank, Murray, UT 84107, USA
4. School of Medicine, University of Utah, Salt Lake City, UT 84132, USA
5. Brigham Young University, Provo, UT 84602, USA
6. College of Osteopathic Medicine, Rocky Vista University, Ivins, UT 80112, USA
* Correspondence: cornea2020@me.com; Tel.: +1-801-568-0200

Abstract: The purpose of this study was to compare the accuracy of several intraocular (IOL) lens power calculation formulas in long eyes. This was a single-site retrospective consecutive case series that reviewed patients with axial lengths (AL) > 28.0 mm who underwent phacoemulsification. The Wang–Koch (WK) adjustment and Cooke-modified axial length (CMAL) adjustment were applied to Holladay 1 and SRK/T. The median absolute error (MedAE) and the percentage of eyes with prediction errors ±0.25 diopters (D), ±0.50 D, ±0.75 D, and ±1.00 D were used to analyze the formula's accuracy. This study comprised a total of 35 eyes from 25 patients. The Kane formula had the lowest MedAE of all the formulas, but all were comparable except Holladay 1, which had a significantly lower prediction accuracy with either AL adjustment. The SRK/T formula with the CMAL adjustment had the highest accuracy in predicting the formula outcome within ±0.50 D. The newer formulas (BU-II, EVO, Hill-RBF version 3.0, and Kane) were all equally predictable in long eyes. The SRK/T formula with the CMAL adjustment was comparable to these newer formulas with better outcomes than the WK adjustment. The Holladay 1 with either AL adjustment had the lowest predictive accuracy.

Keywords: IOL accuracy; high myope; high axial length; Caucasian; Kane; Barrett; EVO; Hill-RBF; Holladay 1; SRK/T

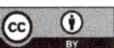

1. Introduction

The accurate calculation of intraocular lens (IOL) power is critical for providing optimal visual acuity results for cataract surgery patients. As axial lengths reach the extremes, the variation in outcomes increases significantly, demonstrating the need to carefully select the best formula [1–3]. The first-generation SRK I, second-generation SRK II, and Hoffer formulas have given way to the more modern third-generation Holladay 1, Hoffer Q, and SRK/T formulas, as well as the fourth-generation Haigis and Barrett Universal II (BU-II) formulas [3,4]. The SRK/T formula, in particular, has been shown to be particularly accurate in eyes with an AL ≥ 27.0 mm [5–7]. More recent formulas include the Hill–Radial Basis Function version 3.0, Emmetropia Verifying Optical (EVO), and Kane [7–9]. The resulting improvement in accuracy has increased the popularity of newer formulas among cataract surgeons [1,5,10].

Despite the increased accuracy of the newer third- and fourth-generation formulas, they tend to underestimate IOL power for patients with longer eyes, causing postoperative hyperopia [11]. An AL modification method, referred to as the Wang–Koch (WK) adjustment, was published by Wang et al. in 2017, which increases the accuracy of older generation formulas in patients with high AL [11]. Fernández et al. demonstrated that the variation in prediction error (PE) with axial length was due to considering a single refractive index and not due to errors in the prediction of effective lens position (ELP), suggesting a variation in the fictitious refractive index to address this problem [12]. In 2019, the Cooke-modified axial length (CMAL) method was proposed, which sums the individual ocular segment lengths to predict a sum-of-segments AL that improved the predictive power of third- and fourth-generation formulas in long and short eyes [13]. The addition of these methods increased the prediction accuracy of newer generation formulas such as SRK/T and Holladay in highly myopic eyes [5,14].

The BU-II formula was first presented as a modified version of the original Barrett formula in 2010; it is considered one of the most accurate but remains unpublished [5,9]. Other unpublished formulas include the EVO (Tun Kuan Yeo, MD), Kane (Jack Kane, MD), and Hill-RBF version 3.0 [9,15]. The Kane and Hill-RBF version 3.0 formulas both incorporate artificial intelligence to predict IOL power [7]. The newly updated Hill-RBF version 3.0 increased the database for eyes of all sizes, including myopic patients, and added central corneal thickness (CCT), lens thickness (LT), white-to-white (WTW), and gender to the existing parameters [15].

To our knowledge, the vast majority of studies evaluating the accuracy of the newer formulas in highly myopic patients have taken place with Asian participants, where high myopia is more common [16,17]. As eyes in Asian populations also tend to have flatter corneas, it is possible that the use of these formulas in other racial groups with longer axial lengths could have differing results [18,19]. Given this paucity of data outside of Asian populations, there is a need for studies of these newer formulas in highly myopic patients of non-Asian descent. The purpose of this study was to compare the IOL accuracy of six IOL power formulas for eyes with extremely long axial lengths ($\geq$28.0 mm) from a predominantly Caucasian population.

2. Materials and Methods

2.1. Subjects and Procedures

This study was a retrospective review of consecutive cataract patients having undergone uncomplicated phacoemulsification procedures at a single site from January 2013 to May 2021. The Lenstar® LS 900 (Haag-Streit AG, Koeniz, Switzerland) reviewed 16,538 eyes and initially identified 71 records of patients with axial lengths > 28.0 mm who subsequently underwent simple phacoemulsification. Patients included had a manifest refraction performed at least one month postoperatively with a corrected distance visual acuity (CDVA) of 20/40 or better. Eyes with prior refractive surgery, intraoperative or postoperative cataract complications, a history of severe fundus pathology (e.g., myopic degeneration or macular hole), or a lack of postoperative refraction at one month or greater were excluded; this left 35 eyes of 25 patients for analysis (Figure S1). The data were de-identified prior to analysis.

Biometric measurements included AL, keratometry (K), anterior chamber depth (ACD, measured from the corneal epithelium to the lens), WTW, CCT, LT, and aqueous depth. Preoperative refraction, uncorrected distance visual acuity (UDVA), and CDVA were noted as well. All visual acuity measurements were converted to the equivalent logarithm of the minimum angle of resolution (LogMAR). Additionally, the patient's age, gender, and past ocular and medical history were included in the data analysis. The patient's self-reported ethnicity data were not recorded in the paper charts. Ethnicity was projected from the area's demographics and recent census data.

2.2. Surgery and Intraocular Lenses

The standard phacoemulsification procedure was performed on all the patients by a single experienced surgeon using topical anesthesia. One of six different foldable acrylic lenses was inserted into the eye. The models of IOL lens choices included the AR40e (Sensar®, Johnson & Johnson Vision, Jacksonville, FL, USA), MA60MA (Alcon Laboratories, Fort Worth, TX, USA), MX60E (enVista®, Bausch + Lomb, Rochester, NY, USA), ZCB00 (TECNIS®, Johnson & Johnson Vision, Jacksonville, FL, USA), ZCT225 (TECNIS®, Johnson

& Johnson Vision, Jacksonville, FL, USA), and ZXR00 (TECNIS Symfony®, Johnson & Johnson Vision, Jacksonville, FL, USA). Patients were instructed to use third- or fourth-generation fluoroquinolone antibiotic eye drops four times daily for one week. Patients were also started on a topical steroid medication four times daily and tapered weekly over one month. A topical NSAID eye drop was used twice daily for six weeks. Patients were then scheduled for one-day, one-week, and one-month follow-up appointments where the LogMAR, UDVA, and intraocular pressure (IOP) were checked. At the one-month postoperative appointment, manifest refraction was performed, and LogMAR CDVA was recorded. Any additional follow-up appointments were recorded within two years; IOP, CDVA, UDVA, and manifest refractions were recorded for any of these follow-up visits. The last manifest refraction charted was recorded as the patient's postoperative spherical equivalent (SE) to analyze the prediction error.

2.3. Retrospective and Statistical Analysis

The six formulas evaluated were:

(1) Barrett Universal II (available at https://calc.apacrs.org/barrett_universal2105/, hereafter referred to as BU-II, accessed 12 September 2021);
(2) Emmetropia Verifying Optical (available at https://www.evoiolcalculator.com/, referred to as EVO, accessed 12 September 2021);
(3) Hill–Radial Bias Function 3.0 Calculator (available at https://rbfcalculator.com/, hereafter referred to as Hill-RBF, accessed 12 September 2021);
(4) Holladay 1 [20];
(5) Kane (available at https://www.iolformula.com/, accessed 12 September 2021);
(6) SRK/T [21].

Due to the small study sample and evaluation of long eyes, IOL constants for the implanted lenses were obtained from those listed in the User Group for Laser Interference Biometry database (available at http://ocusoft.de/ulib/c1.htm, referred to as ULIB, accessed 15 June 2021). To calculate the predicted SEs, the ULIB IOL constants for each lens and the patient's biometric data were input into each formula. The published Holladay 1 and SRK/T formulas were exported directly into Excel (Microsoft Corporation, Redmond, WA, USA). The AL was adjusted for the Holladay 1 and SRK/T formulas using the modified regression WK adjustment and the CMAL adjustment, resulting in two iterations of each formula. For the remaining four unpublished formulas, ULIB IOL constants and biometrics were input into the online calculators via Python (Python Software Foundation, Wilmington, DE, USA) as recommended by Hoffer and Savini [22]. Refractive prediction errors (PE) were then calculated by subtracting the formula-predicted SE refractive error from the postoperative manifest refraction SE. Absolute prediction errors (AE) were calculated from the PE.

Mean prediction error (MPE) was used to assess for postoperative myopic or hyperopic surprises. As described by Hoffer and Savini, the mean absolute error (MAE) and median absolute error (MedAE) were calculated for each formula to assess the predictive accuracy [22]. The max AE was noted for each formula as well. The cases were analyzed by the percentage of eyes with a PE of ±0.25 diopters (D), ±0.50 D, ±0.75 D, and ±1.00 D for each formula. The postop refraction values were rounded to the closest step to account for the invariant refraction assumption.

Statistical analysis was performed using R version 4.0.2 (22 June 2020) statistical software. Continuous variables were reported with a mean and standard deviation (SD), and categorical variables were reported with a number and percentage. The normality of the data was assessed with the Shapiro–Wilk test. The distribution of the AE values did not follow normal Gaussian distribution, so nonparametric tests were used. The difference in refractive errors between formulas was assessed with the paired Wilcoxon signed-rank test. The percentages of PE within ±0.25 D, ±0.50 D, ±0.75 D, and ±1.00 D for each formula were compared with a Cochran's Q test. McNemar's test with Bonferroni adjustment was then used to identify any statistically significant difference identified in the Cochran's Q. A p-value less than 0.05 was considered statistically significant.

3. Results

3.1. Population Demographics

The study comprised 35 eyes of 25 patients. The mean age of the study was 56.94 ± 9.56 years and 60% of the patients were female. The mean axial length was 28.71 ± 0.87 mm (range: 28.01 mm to 31.10 mm). The mean corneal power was 43.30 ± 1.61 D, with the majority of patients' average keratometry (65.7%) falling between 42.0 D and 46.0 D. The average ACD was 3.66 ± 0.38 mm and the average LT of the patient was 4.25 ± 0.52 mm. Table 1 summarizes all the biometrics, refractive outcomes, and demographics of the study population.

Table 1. Demographics, biometrics, and refractive outcomes (n = 35).

	n	(%)
Gender (F/M)	15/10	(60.0%, 40.0%)
Eye (OD/OS)	20/15	(57.1%, 42.9%)

	Mean ± SD	Range
Age, y	56.94 ± 9.56	37, 76
Axial length (mm)	28.71 ± 0.87	28.01, 31.1
ACD (mm)	3.66 ± 0.38	2.38, 4.24
Lens thickness (mm)	4.25 ± 0.52	2.96, 5.6
Average keratometry (D)	43.30 ± 1.61	41.59, 49.22

	n	(%)
Keratometry subgroups		
Flat (<42.0 D)	10	(28.6%)
Medium (42.0 D–46.0 D)	23	(65.7%)
Steep (>46.0 D)	2	(5.7%)
IOL Type		
Alcon MA60MA	2	(5.7%)
AMO AR40e	2	(5.7%)
enVista MX60E	1	(2.9%)
Tecnis ZCB00	24	(68.6%)
Tecnis ZCT225	2	(5.7%)
Tecnis ZXR00	4	(11.4%)

	Mean ± SD	Range
IOL power (D)	7.76 ± 3.06	−1.00, +12.00
Preoperative		
SE (D)	−11.28 ± 4.29	−18.88, −3.63
UDVA (LogMAR)	1.69 ± 0.39	0.3, 1.90
CDVA (LogMAR)	0.22 ± 0.17	0, 1.00
Postoperative		
SE (D)	−0.58 ± 0.79	−2.13, 0.75
UDVA (LogMAR)	0.20 ± 0.23	0, 0.80
CDVA (LogMAR)	0.01 ± 0.07	−0.12, 0.30
Postoperative refraction, days after surgery	147.62 ± 179.90	21, 686

D = diopters; F = female; IOL = intraocular; M = male; mm = millimeters; OD = right eye; OS = left eye; SD = standard deviation.

The refractive measurements show a marked improvement in refractive error following phacoemulsification surgery. The mean CDVA before the procedure was 0.22 ± 0.17 (LogMAR) and improved to 0.01 ± 0.07 (LogMAR) after the procedure. After surgery, the mean SE approached emmetropia at −0.58 ± 0.79 compared to a mean preoperative SE that was highly myopic at −11.28 ± 4.29. The implanted IOLs had a mean power of 7.76 ± 3.06 D (range: −1.00 to +12.00 D) with only one (2.86%) implanted lens with a minus power diopter (Table 1).

3.2. Accuracy of the Six Formulas

Figure 1A shows the distribution and interquartile ranges of the PEs for each formula, and Table 2 shows the MPE of each formula to illustrate the tendency of each formula to lead to either myopic or hyperopic surprises. The four newer formulas tended to result in hyperopic surprises as compared with the older SRK/T and Holladay 1 formulas. The WK AL adjustment tended to lead to a myopic surprise for both SRK/T and Holladay 1. In contrast, the CMAL adjustment tended towards a hyperopic shift for Holladay 1. Interestingly, the median value of PE closest to zero was the SRK/T formula with CMAL adjustment, and this formula's MPE is also closest to zero. Kane's formula had the lowest MedAE (0.270), with the three newer formulas (BU-II, EVO, and Hill-RBF) following closely behind (Table 2). The WK adjustment, with either SRK/T or Holladay 1, had the highest MedAE values. The WK adjustment for SRK/T had the highest MedAE of all the formulas, but the CMAL adjustment with SRK/T was not far from the BU-II formula. The Wilcoxon signed-rank test revealed a statistically significant difference ($p < 0.05$) of the WK adjustment to either SRK/T and Holladay 1 compared to the CMAL adjustment of SRK/T, indicating that the WK adjustment, with either formula, had lower accuracy (Table 3). Figure 1B shows a boxplot of the AEs for each formula. The Holladay 1 with WK adjustment and SRK/T with WK adjustment had the widest range and highest MedAE compared with the CMAL adjustments or the four newer formulas.

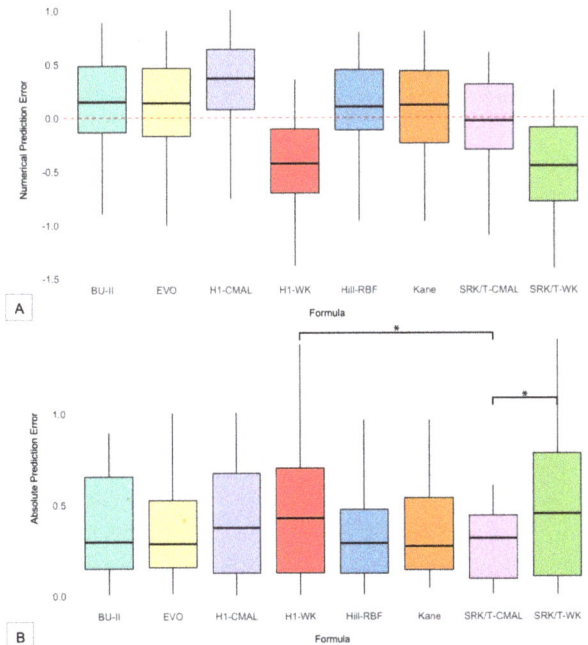

Figure 1. Boxplots showing the prediction errors of intraocular lens calculation formulas. (**A**) The numerical prediction errors were calculated by subtracting the predicted spherical equivalent (SE) from the postoperative SE. (**B**) The absolute prediction errors were then taken from the numerical prediction errors. BU-II = Barrett Universal II; CMAL = Cooke-modified axial length; EVO = Emmetropia Verifying Optical; H1 = Holladay 1; WK = Wang–Koch AL adjustment. * significant $p < 0.05$.

Table 2. Comparison of predictive outcomes.

Formula	MPE	SD	MAE	MedAE	Max AE	± 0.25 D [a]	± 0.50 D [a]	± 0.75 D [a]	± 1.00 D [a]
BU-II	0.146	0.451	0.379	0.295	0.895	45.71	68.57	85.71	100.00
EVO	0.147	0.416	0.361	0.285	1.005	42.86	71.43	91.43	97.14
Hill-RBF	0.136	0.407	0.333	0.288	0.965	47.06	76.47	91.18	100.00
H1-CMAL	0.352	0.393	0.419	0.370	1.010	40.00	57.14	77.14	94.29
H1-WK	−0.396	0.401	0.450	0.430	1.380	37.14	57.14	80.00	94.29
Kane	0.082	0.418	0.346	0.270	0.810	42.86	68.57	91.43	100.00
SRK/T-CMAL	−0.015	0.385	0.303	0.310	1.100	45.45	87.88	96.97	96.97
SRK/T-WK	−0.442	0.411	0.474	0.450	1.410	33.33	54.45	69.70	93.94

AE = absolute prediction error; BU-II = Barrett Universal II; CMAL = Cooke-modified axial length; D = diopters; EVO = Emmetropia Verifying Optical; H1 = Holladay 1; MAE = mean absolute prediction error; MedAE = median absolute prediction error; MPE = mean numerical prediction error; Max AE = maximum absolute prediction error SD = standard deviation; WK = Wang–Koch axial length adjustment. a = % of patients with refractive prediction errors within 0.25 D, 0.50 D, 0.75 D, or 1.00 D.

Table 3. Statistical analysis comparison of AE.

Formulas	BU-II	EVO	Hill-RBF	H1-CMAL	H1-WK	Kane	SRK/T-CMAL	SRK/T-WK
BU-II	-	-	-	-	-	-	-	-
EVO	0.762	-	-	-	-	-	-	-
Hill-RBF	0.189	0.442	-	-	-	-	-	-
H1-CMAL	0.09	0.114	0.097	-	-	-	-	-
H1-WK	0.408	0.207	0.156	0.801	-	-	-	-
Kane	0.158	0.172	0.974	0.073	0.164	-	-	-
SRK/T-CMAL	0.073	0.153	0.562	0.125	0.012 [†]	0.376	-	-
SRK/T-WK	0.331	0.161	0.200	0.514	0.335	0.153	0.010 [†]	-

AE = absolute prediction errors; BU-II = Barrett Universal II; CMAL = Cooke-modified axial length; EVO = Emmetropia Verifying Optical; H1 = Holladay 1; WK = Wang–Koch axial length adjustment. † = $p < 0.05$.

Cochran's Q test evaluated the percentage of eyes within ±0.25 D, ±0.50 D, ±0.75 D, and ±1.00 D. The percentages for each formula are stated in Table 2 and graphically represented in Figure 2. The only significant difference among the formulas was found between the percentage of eyes within ±0.50 D and ±0.75 D. Further testing identified that the statistically significant difference was between the SRK/T-CMAL formula compared to the SRK/T-WK, Holladay 1-CMAL, and Holladay 1-WK formulas for the percentage of eyes within ±0.50 D ($p < 0.05$) with SRK/T-CMAL having the highest percentage of eyes with predicted SE within ±0.50 D. The Hill-RBF formula had more accuracy in predicting eyes within ±0.50 D compared with the Holladay 1 with CMAL adjustment ($p = 0.0143$). When assessing the percentage of eyes that achieved postoperative refraction within 0.75 D of the predicted SE, the SRK/T with WK adjustment did significantly worse than the remaining formulas ($p < 0.05$) with only the exception of the Holladay 1 with WK adjustment formula, which performed as poorly as the SRK/T-WK. The BU-II, Hill-RBF, and Kane formulas could predict the postoperative manifest refraction within 1.00 D for all 35 eyes.

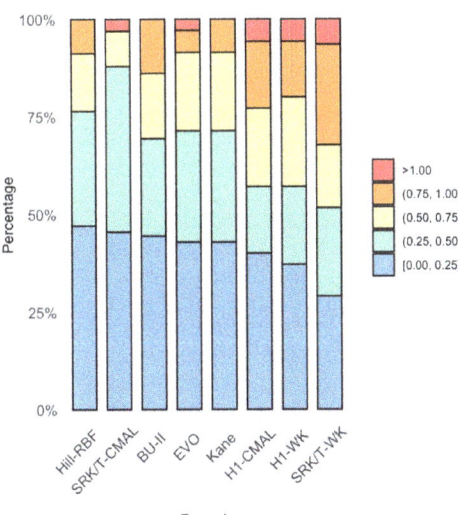

Figure 2. Stacked histogram comparing the percentage of eyes within ±0.25 diopters (D), ±0.50 D, ±0.75 D, and ±1.00 D of predicted spherical equivalent for various intraocular lens calculation formulas. BU-II = Barrett Universal II; CMAL = Cooke-modified axial length; EVO = Emmetropia verifying optical; H1 = Holladay 1; WK = Wang–Koch AL adjustment.

4. Discussion

In this study, we assessed the accuracy of BU-II, EVO, Hill-RBF, Holladay 1, Kane, and SRK/T in long eyes in a predominantly Caucasian population. Despite advances in formulas, surgeons are still faced with the difficulty of accurately achieving desired refractive outcomes for high myopes. In our study, the newer-generation BU-II, EVO, Hill-RBF 3.0, and Kane formulas had greater accuracy than the third-generation Holladay 1 formula with either the WK or CMAL adjustment. The SRK/T with CMAL adjustment was comparable to the newer IOL formulas. The WK axial length adjustment for SRK/T did not prove to be as accurate as the CMAL adjustment and was comparable to the accuracy of Holladay 1 (Figure 1 and Table 2).

Asians have a higher percentage of high myopia as compared with Caucasians [16,17]. As a result, most studies assessing IOL calculation accuracy within high AL have been performed in predominantly Asian study populations [14,23–32]. While our study did not have ethnicity data readily available in the paper charts, the population demographics of the study site (Draper, UT) are 91.1% white and 3.5% Asian (US Census Data for Draper, UT, available at https://www.census.gov/quickfacts/drapercityutah, accessed 27 June 2021). To the surgeon's knowledge, only one patient was of Asian descent in the study. There have been fewer studies assessing IOL formula accuracy evaluating AL greater than 25.0 mm in predominantly Caucasian populations, and even fewer evaluating the newer vergence or artificial intelligence formulas [33–35]. The criteria for these studies were AL >25.0, 26.0, or 26.5 mm, whereas the current study evaluated much longer eyes. In addition to having a higher percentage of eyes with longer ALs, some studies have shown that Asians have flatter corneal shapes as compared with Caucasians [18,19]. Axial length and corneal shape are two variables known to heavily influence the predictive capabilities of IOL formulas [27].

Assessing the accuracy of the formulas, the MedAE of the four newer formulas, Hill-RBF, Kane, EVO, and BU-II, had the lowest prediction errors, with Kane having the lowest of all the formulas and BU-II coming in fourth. The only significant difference in MedAE identified between formulas was the Holladay 1 formula with the CMAL adjustment, which performed significantly worse than any of the four newer formulas or the SRK/T with CMAL adjustment (Table 2 and Figure 1). Similarly, in assessing the percentage of eyes that achieved a prediction error of ±0.25 D, ±0.50 D, ±0.75 D, or ±1.00 D, BU-II, Hill-RBF, EVO Kane, and SRK/T-CMAL had the highest percentage of eyes within 0.25 D. The statistical difference showed that SRK/T-CMAL had a higher accuracy of predicting SE within 0.50 D than the Holladay 1 formulas and the WK adjustment of SRK/T. The Holladay 1 formula with WK adjustment did worse than the other remaining formulas in predicting the SE ±0.75 D (Table 2). The four new formulas also tended to predict postoperative hyperopic shift compared with the older formulas, which tended to predict a postoperative myopic shift. This result is consistent with the previous studies that have documented the tendency for newer fourth-generation formulas to lead to postoperative hyperopia as compared with older-generation formulas, which tend to have greater postoperative myopia [11].

A similar study compared the same formulas as the current study, except that they used version 2.0 of the Hill-RBF formula and looked at a population of 370 high-AL eyes of a predominantly Asian population [32]. Their study showed that the Holladay 1 with WK adjustment and Kane formulas had higher accuracy in extremely high myopes. Of note their study defined extreme myopia as AL ≥ 30.0 mm, while the current study only had four patients that fit this criterion. However, Fuest et al. in Germany looked at eyes with long axial lengths and compared the BU-II and Hill-RBF 2.0 with Holladay 1 and SRK/T formulas and found that the BU-II and Hill-RBF 2.0 performed better than the Holladay 1 and SRK/T formulas, which was consistent with other studies, including studies consisting of Asian populations [1,34–37]. Our data support previous reports that the BU-II and Hill-RBF perform more accurately than Holladay 1 and SRK/T in long eyes. This study was able to add that the Kane, EVO, and SRK/T-CMAL formulas performed similarly to BU-II and Hill-RBF in predominately Caucasian eyes. Similar studies in four Asian populations and one European population also found newer-generation formulas such as the Kane EVO, and BU-II to be most accurate in long eyes [38–42].

Our study did have some limitations: (1) Because very high axial lengths are less frequent in the population and even less so in Caucasian populations, our study sample size was not as robust as other Asian studies, and we included bilateral eyes as a result of the small size. The use of bilateral eyes can potentially compound data. (2) The chart data did not include the patient's self-reported ethnicity, and therefore assumptions were made based on the demographics of the location of the surgical center and the physician's recollection of presumed ethnicity. (3) The study was retrospective and we had limitations in standardization and follow-up periods. Future studies on larger sample sizes of Caucasian populations or a single-site comparison of Asian to Caucasian would be warranted.

In conclusion, our results show that for axial lengths greater than or equal to 28.0 mm, the Barrett Universal II, Emmetropia Verifying Optical, Hill-RBF version 3.0, and Kane formulas were comparable in accuracy. Additionally, the Cooke-modified axial length adjustment was better than the Wang–Koch axial length adjustment when used with the SRK/T formula. The Holladay 1 had the lowest predictive accuracy of the six formulas we tested. The most accurate prediction of high axial lengths in Caucasian eyes may be achieved with Barrett Universal II, Emmetropia Verifying Optical, Hill-RBF version 3.0, Kane, and SRK/T with the CMAL adjustment.

Supplementary Materials: The following supporting information can be downloaded at: https://www.mdpi.com/article/10.3390/jcm11195947/s1, **Figure S1**: Flow diagram illustrates the process by which patients were selected for the study to obtain the predicted postoperative spherical equivalent (SE) used to analyze the prediction accuracy of the six formulas. The axial lengths were modified with the Wang–Koch and Cooke-modified adjustment prior to their input in the Holladay 1 and SRK/T formulas. The Barrett Universal II, Kane, Emmetropia Verifying Optical (EVO), and Hill-RBF version 3.0 formulas are all unpublished, and the biometric data were input directly into their respective online calculators.

Author Contributions: Conceptualization, M.M.; methodology, M.M.; formal analysis, K.M.D. and D.P.B.; resources, P.C.H.; data curation, K.M.D., T.S.P. and I.M.D.; writing—original draft preparation, K.M.D., J.L.J., M.M., D.P.B. and T.S.P.; writing—review and editing, K.M.D., J.L.J., M.M. and Y.C.R.; supervision, M.M., Y.C.R. and P.C.H.; project administration, P.C.H.; funding acquisition, M.M. All authors have read and agreed to the published version of the manuscript.

Funding: This study was funded by an unrestricted grant from Research to Prevent Blindness (RPB), 360 Lexington Avenue, 22nd Floor New York, NY 10017. No support was received for the publication of this article.

Institutional Review Board Statement: The study was conducted in accordance with the Declaration of Helsinki and approved by the Institutional Review Board of the Biomedical Research Alliance of New York (BRANY, protocol 20-12-547-823). This study was approved by the Hoopes Vision Ethics Board and was HIPAA-compliant.

Informed Consent Statement: Informed consent was obtained from all subjects involved in the study.

Data Availability Statement: The data presented are available upon request to the corresponding author. The data are not publicly available due to patient privacy.

Acknowledgments: We thank Shannon McCabe who provided guidance, expertise, and constructive criticism of the manuscript.

Conflicts of Interest: The authors declare no conflict of interest. The funders had no role in the design of the study; in the collection, analyses, or interpretation of data; in the writing of the manuscript; or in the decision to publish the results.

References

1. Melles, R.B.; Holladay, J.T.; Chang, W.J. Accuracy of Intraocular Lens Calculation Formulas. *Ophthalmology* **2018**, *125*, 169–178. [CrossRef]
2. Davis, G. The Evolution of Cataract Surgery. *Mo. Med.* **2016**, *113*, 58. [CrossRef]
3. Doshi, D.; Limdi, P.; Parekh, N.; Gohil, N. A Comparative Study to Assess the Predictability of Different IOL Power Calculation Formulas in Eyes of Short and Long Axial Length. *J. Clin. Diagn. Res.* **2017**, *11*, NC01–NC04. [CrossRef] [PubMed]
4. Amro, M.; Chanbour, W.; Arej, N.; Jarade, E. Third- and fourth-generation formulas for intraocular lens power calculation before and after phakic intraocular lens insertion in high myopia. *J. Cataract Refract. Surg.* **2018**, *44*, 1321–1325. [CrossRef]
5. Kuthirummal, N.; Vanathi, M.; Mukhija, R.; Gupta, N.; Meel, R.; Saxena, R.; Tandon, R. Evaluation of Barrett universal II formula for intraocular lens power calculation in Asian Indian population. *Indian J. Ophthalmol.* **2020**, *68*, 59–64. [CrossRef]
6. Aristodemou, P.; Cartwright, N.E.K.; Sparrow, J.M.; Johnston, R.L. Formula choice: Hoffer Q, Holladay 1, or SRK/T and refractive outcomes in 8108 eyes after cataract surgery with biometry by partial coherence interferometry. *J. Cataract Refract. Surg.* **2011**, *37*, 63–71. [CrossRef]
7. Xia, T.; Martinez, C.E.; Tsai, L.M. Update on Intraocular Lens Formulas and Calculations. *Asia-Pacific J. Ophthalmol.* **2020**, *9*, 186–193. [CrossRef]
8. Kane, J.X.; Van Heerden, A.; Atik, A.; Petsoglou, C. Accuracy of 3 new methods for intraocular lens power selection. *J. Cataract Refract. Surg.* **2017**, *43*, 333–339. [CrossRef]
9. Savini, G.; Hoffer, K.J.; Balducci, N.; Barboni, P.; Schiano-Lomoriello, D. Comparison of formula accuracy for intraocular lens power calculation based on measurements by a swept-source optical coherence tomography optical biometer. *J. Cataract. Refract. Surg.* **2020**, *46*, 27–33. [PubMed]
10. Turnbull, A.M.; Hill, W.E.; Barrett, G.D. Accuracy of intraocular lens power calculation methods when targeting low myopia in monovision. *J. Cataract Refract. Surg.* **2020**, *46*, 862–866. [CrossRef]
11. Wang, L.; Shirayama, M.; Ma, X.J.; Kohnen, T.; Koch, D.D. Optimizing intraocular lens power calculations in eyes with axial lengths above 25.0 mm. *J. Cataract Refract. Surg.* **2011**, *37*, 2018–2027. [CrossRef]
12. Fernández, J.; Rodríguez-Vallejo, M.; Martínez, J.; Tauste, A.; Piñero, D.P. New Approach for the Calculation of the Intraocular Lens Power Based on the Fictitious Corneal Refractive Index Estimation. *J. Ophthalmol.* **2019**, *2019*, 279612. [CrossRef] [PubMed]
13. Cooke, D.L.; Cooke, T.L. Approximating sum-of-segments axial length from a traditional optical low-coherence reflectometry measurement. *J. Cataract Refract. Surg.* **2019**, *45*, 351–354. [CrossRef]
14. Zhang, J.; Tan, X.; Wang, W.; Yang, G.; Xu, J.; Ruan, X.; Gu, X.; Luo, L. Effect of Axial Length Adjustment Methods on Intraocular Lens Power Calculation in Highly Myopic Eyes. *Am. J. Ophthalmol.* **2020**, *214*, 110–118. [CrossRef] [PubMed]
15. Tsessler, M.; Cohen, S.; Wang, L.; Koch, D.D.; Zadok, D.; Abulafia, A. Evaluating the prediction accuracy of the Hill-RBF 3.0 formula using a heteroscedastic statistical method. *J. Cataract Refract. Surg.* **2021**, *48*, 37–43. [CrossRef]
16. Hoffer, K.J.; Savini, G. Effect of Gender and Race on Ocular Biometry. *Int. Ophthalmol. Clin.* **2017**, *57*, 137–142. [CrossRef]
17. Ikuno, Y. Overview of the complications of high myopia. *Retina* **2017**, *37*, 2347–2351. [CrossRef]

18. Lin, M.C.; Chen, Y.Q.; Polse, K.A. The Effects of Ocular and Lens Parameters on the Postlens Tear Thickness. *Eye Contact Lens: Sci. Clin. Pract.* **2003**, *29* (Suppl. S1), S33–S36. [CrossRef] [PubMed]
19. Hickson-Curran, S.; Young, G.; Brennan, N.; Hunt, C. Chinese and Caucasian ocular topography and soft contact lens fit. *Clin. Exp. Optom.* **2016**, *99*, 149–156. [CrossRef]
20. Holladay, J.T.; Musgrove, K.H.; Prager, T.C.; Lewis, J.W.; Chandler, T.Y.; Ruiz, R.S. A three-part system for refining intraocular lens power calculations. *J. Cataract Refract. Surg.* **1988**, *14*, 17–24. [CrossRef]
21. Retzlaff, J.A.; Sanders, D.R.; Kraff, M.C. Development of the SRK/T intraocular lens implant power calculation formula. *J. Cataract Refract. Surg.* **1990**, *16*, 333–340. [CrossRef]
22. Hoffer, K.J.; Savini, G. Update on Intraocular Lens Power Calculation Study Protocols: The Better Way to Design and Report Clinical Trials. *Ophthalmology* **2020**, *128*, e115–e120. [CrossRef] [PubMed]
23. Tsang, C.S.; Chong, G.S.; Yiu, E.P.; Ho, C.K. Intraocular lens power calculation formulas in Chinese eyes with high axial myopia. *J. Cataract Refract. Surg.* **2003**, *29*, 1358–1364. [CrossRef]
24. Wang, J.-K.; Hu, C.-Y.; Chang, S.-W. Intraocular lens power calculation using the IOLMaster and various formulas in eyes with long axial length. *J. Cataract Refract. Surg.* **2008**, *34*, 262–267. [CrossRef] [PubMed]
25. Chen, C.; Xu, X.; Miao, Y.; Zheng, G.; Sun, Y.; Xu, X. Accuracy of Intraocular Lens Power Formulas Involving 148 Eyes with Long Axial Lengths: A Retrospective Chart-Review Study. *J. Ophthalmol.* **2015**, *2015*, 976847. [CrossRef] [PubMed]
26. Zhang, Y.; Liang, X.Y.; Liu, S.; Lee, J.W.Y.; Bhaskar, S.; Lam, D.S.C. Accuracy of Intraocular Lens Power Calculation Formulas for Highly Myopic Eyes. *J. Ophthalmol.* **2016**, *2016*, 1917268. [CrossRef]
27. Zhang, Z.; Miao, Y.; Fang, X.; Luo, Q.; Wang, Y. Accuracy of the Haigis and SRK/T Formulas in Eyes Longer than 29.0 mm and the Influence of Central Corneal Keratometry Reading. *Curr. Eye Res.* **2018**, *43*, 1316–1321. [CrossRef]
28. Rong, X.; He, W.; Zhu, Q.; Qian, D.; Lu, Y.; Zhu, X. Intraocular lens power calculation in eyes with extreme myopia: Comparison of Barrett Universal II, Haigis, and Olsen formulas. *J. Cataract Refract. Surg.* **2019**, *45*, 732–737. [CrossRef]
29. Wan, K.H.; Lam, T.C.; Yu, M.C.; Chan, T.C. Accuracy and Precision of Intraocular Lens Calculations Using the New Hill-RBF Version 2.0 in Eyes With High Axial Myopia. *Am. J. Ophthalmol.* **2019**, *205*, 66–73. [CrossRef]
30. Deng, G.; Zhou, D.; Sun, Z. Accuracy of the refractive prediction determined by intraocular lens power calculation formulas in high myopia. *Indian J. Ophthalmol.* **2019**, *67*, 484–489. [CrossRef]
31. Zhang, J.-Q.; Zou, X.-Y.; Zheng, D.-Y.; Chen, W.-R.; Sun, A.; Luo, L.-X. Effect of lens constants optimization on the accuracy of intraocular lens power calculation formulas for highly myopic eyes. *Int. J. Ophthalmol.* **2019**, *12*, 943–948. [CrossRef] [PubMed]
32. Cheng, H.; Wang, L.; Kane, J.X.; Liangping, L.; Liu, L.; Wu, M. Accuracy of Artificial Intelligence Formulas and Axial Length Adjustments for Highly Myopic Eyes. *Am. J. Ophthalmol.* **2020**, *223*, 100–107. [CrossRef] [PubMed]
33. Tang, K.S.; Tran, E.M.; Chen, A.J.; Rivera, D.R.; Rivera, J.J.; Greenberg, P.B. Accuracy of biometric formulae for intraocular lens power calculation in a teaching hospital. *Int. J. Ophthalmol.* **2020**, *13*, 61–65. [CrossRef] [PubMed]
34. Roessler, G.F.; Dietlein, T.S.; Plange, N.; Roepke, A.-K.; Dinslage, S.; Walter, P.; Mazinani, B.A. Accuracy of intraocular lens power calculation using partial coherence interferometry in patients with high myopia. *Ophthalmic Physiol. Opt.* **2012**, *32*, 228–233. [CrossRef]
35. Fuest, M.; Plange, N.; Kuerten, D.; Schellhase, H.; Mazinani, B.A.E.; Walter, P.; Kohnen, S.; Widder, R.A.; Roessler, G. Intraocular lens power calculation for plus and minus lenses in high myopia using partial coherence interferometry. *Int. Ophthalmol.* **2021**, *41*, 1585–1592. [CrossRef]
36. Ji, J.; Liu, Y.; Zhang, J.; Wu, X.; Shao, W.; Ma, B.; Luo, M. Comparison of six methods for the intraocular lens power calculation in high myopic eyes. *Eur. J. Ophthalmol.* **2019**, *31*, 96–102. [CrossRef] [PubMed]
37. Chang, P.; Qian, S.; Wang, Y.; Li, S.; Yang, F.; Hu, Y.; Liu, Z.; Zhao, Y.-E. Accuracy of new-generation intraocular lens calculation formulas in eyes with variations in predicted refraction. *Graefe's Arch. Clin. Exp. Ophthalmol.* **2022**, 1–9. [CrossRef]
38. Guo, C.; Yin, S.; Qiu, K.; Zhang, M. Comparison of accuracy of intraocular lens power calculation for eyes with an axial length greater than 29.0 mm. *Int. Ophthalmol.* **2022**, *42*, 2029–2038. [CrossRef]
39. Chu, Y.-C.; Huang, T.-L.; Chang, P.-Y.; Ho, W.-T.; Hsu, Y.-R.; Chang, S.-W.; Wang, J.-K. Predictability of 6 Intraocular Lens Power Calculation Formulas in People With Very High Myopia. *Front. Med.* **2022**, *9*, 762761. [CrossRef]
40. Lin, L.; Xu, M.; Mo, E.; Huang, S.; Qi, X.; Gu, S.; Sun, W.; Su, Q.; Li, J.; Zhao, Y.-E. Accuracy of Newer Generation IOL Power Calculation Formulas in Eyes With High Axial Myopia. *J. Refract. Surg.* **2021**, *37*, 754–758. [CrossRef]
41. Tan, Q.; Lin, D.; Wang, L.; Chen, B.; Tang, Q.; Chen, X.; Chen, M.; Tan, J.; Zhang, J.; Wu, L.; et al. Comparison of IOL Power Calculation Formulas for a Trifocal IOL in Eyes With High Myopia. *J. Refract. Surg.* **2021**, *37*, 538–544. [CrossRef] [PubMed]
42. Bernardes, J.; Raimundo, M.; Lobo, C.; Murta, J.N. A Comparison of Intraocular Lens Power Calculation Formulas in High Myopia. *J. Refract. Surg.* **2021**, *37*, 207–211. [CrossRef] [PubMed]

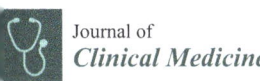

Dry Eye Following Femtosecond Laser-Assisted Cataract Surgery: A Meta-Analysis

Wei-Tsun Chen [1], Yu-Yen Chen [1,2,3,4,5,6,*] and Man-Chen Hung [7]

1. Department of Ophthalmology, Taichung Veterans General Hospital, Taichung 407, Taiwan
2. School of Medicine, National Yang Ming Chiao Tung University, Taipei 112, Taiwan
3. Wilmer Eye Institute, Johns Hopkins University School of Medicine, Baltimore, MD 21287, USA
4. Institute of Public Health and Community Medicine Research Center, National Yang Ming Chiao Tung University, Taipei 112, Taiwan
5. School of Medicine, Chung Shan Medical University, Taichung 402, Taiwan
6. Department of Post-Baccalaureate Medicine, College of Medicine, National Chung Hsing University, Taichung 402, Taiwan
7. Department of Medical Education, Taichung Veterans General Hospital, Taichung 407, Taiwan
* Correspondence: yuyenchen.phd@gmail.com

Abstract: This study investigates the dry eye effect after femtosecond laser-assisted cataract surgery (FLACS) and also compares the risk of postoperative dry eye between FLACS and manual cataract surgery (MCS). We searched various databases between 1 January 2000 and 15 October 2022 and included peer-reviewed clinical studies in our review. Dry eye parameters were extracted at baseline and postoperative day one, week one, one month, and three months. Parameters included were the ocular surface discomfort index (OSDI), tear secretion (tear meniscus height, Schirmer's test), microscopic ocular surface damage (fluorescein staining), and tear stability (first and average tear breakup time). Additionally, the differences of each parameter at each time point were compared between FLACS and MCS. In total, six studies of 611 eyes were included. On postoperative day one, increased, pooled standardised mean differences (SMDs) were noted in the OSDI, tear secretion, tear film instability, and microscopic damage. During postoperative week one, dry eye worsened. Fortunately, dry eye achieved resolution afterwards and nearly returned to the baseline level at postoperative three months. When the parameters were compared between FLACS and MCS, those of FLACS had higher severities, but most were not statistically significant. Dry eye impact was approximately the same in FLACS and MCS at postoperative three months.

Keywords: dry eye; femtosecond laser-assisted cataract surgery (FLACS); phacoemulsification; cornea

1. Introduction

Dry eye is a common postoperative complaint from patients who underwent manual cataract surgery (MCS) with conventional phacoemulsification [1,2]. Symptoms include foreign body sensation, pain, blurred vision, ocular discomfort, burning, and dryness. These symptoms negatively affect patients' satisfaction with surgery, quality of life, and burden public health [3]. After cataract surgery, signs of dry eye include a decreased tear breakup time, decreased corneal sensitivity, and increased ocular surface staining [2,4,5]. The pathogenic factors consist of inflammation, microscopic damage, neurosensory destruction on the ocular surface, tear film instability, and hyperosmolarity [6–8].

Since 2010, the femtosecond laser has been used in cataract surgery. Femtosecond laser-assisted cataract surgery (FLACS) provides precise anterior capsulotomy, safe lens fragmentation, and accurate corneal incision. Thus, it uses less ultrasound energy and phacoemulsification time [9], possibly leading to less postoperative inflammation and less dry eye. However, direct contact of the ocular surface with the vacuum and sustained pressure of the suction ring during FLACS may cause hyperaemia and microscopic damage

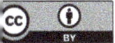

to the ocular surface. In addition, laser procedures in FLACS may potentially affect the tear film [10]. All these reasons may result in dry eye.

Previous studies comparing FLACS and MCS were primarily concerned with the refractory outcome (e.g., visual acuity and spherical equivalent) and complication rate (e.g., anterior capsule tear or posterior capsule rupture) [9,11–16]. However, very few studies have investigated post-FLACS dry eye or compared the risk of dry eye between the two surgery groups. Therefore, we conducted this meta-analysis to investigate the impact of FLACS on dry eye and then compared postoperative dry eye after FLACS and MCS.

2. Materials and Methods

2.1. Search Strategy

This study was conducted according to the preferred reporting items for systematic reviews and meta-analyses (PRISMA) guidelines. We searched the PubMed, EMBASE and Cochrane databases for studies published from 1 January 2000 to 15 October 2022 using the keywords 'femtosecond laser-assisted cataract surgery' and 'dry eye'. Studies were screened first by examining the titles and abstracts and then scrutinising full texts. Bibliographies were also manually searched for the relevant literature.

2.2. Inclusion and Exclusion Criteria

Only peer-reviewed journal articles were included. They should be original, prospective, or randomised control clinical studies investigating dry eye presentation after FLACS. Reviews, meta-analyses, or conference abstracts were excluded because of repeated data. Two researchers (W.-C. Chen and Y.-Y. Chen) independently assessed the articles. A third researcher (M.-C. Hung) intervened if consensus was not reached.

Evaluation of the quality of included articles was performed independently by two researchers (W.-C. Chen and Y.-Y. Chen) using ROBINS-I risk of bias assessment tool. A third researcher (M.-C. Hung) reassessed and made the final decision if discrepancies occurred. ROBINS-I assesses the risk of bias in 7 domains, including confounding, selection of participants, classification of interventions, deviations from intended interventions, missing data, measurement of outcomes, and selection of the reported result. Each domain contains a set of questions (criteria). The risk of bias judgement of each domain was categorised into 'Low risk', 'Moderate risk', 'Serious risk', and 'Critical risk' of bias. Then the overall risk of bias was judged according to the assessment of each domain.

2.3. Data Extraction

The following data were tracked from each included article: the first author, year of publication, and number/age/gender of participants. We also recorded the baseline (preoperative) and postoperative parameters regarding dry eye with: the ocular surface disease index (OSDI), tear meniscus height, Schirmer's test, fluorescein staining, first tear breakup time, and average tear breakup time.

2.4. Definitions of Parameters

The OSDI was adopted to evaluate dry eye symptoms. The questionnaire included 12 questions about eye discomfort, visual function, and environmental triggers. A higher OSDI implies more severe dry eye [17]. Tear meniscus height was assessed via corneal topography in order to measure the height of the inferior tear meniscus [18]. A lower tear meniscus height implies a sign of dry eye. Schirmer's test, also an index of tear secretion, was performed with sterile strips inserted at the lateral third of the lower eyelid margin [19]. The strips were removed five minutes later and the amount of wetting of the paper strips was measured. A lower Schirmer score suggests the diagnosis of dry eye. Fluorescein staining was applied to assess ocular surface damage [20]. Topical fluorescein readily enters and stains the corneal stroma where the epithelium is absent or when the epithelial cells have lost intercellular junctions. A higher score of fluorescein staining is a sign of dry eye. Tear film breakup time is a clinical evaluation of evaporative dry eye disease. Further, it is performed by instilling topical fluorescein into the eyes [21]. The number of seconds that elapsed between the last blink and the appearance of the first dry spot in the tear film was recorded as the first tear breakup time. Similarly, the average tear breakup time was recorded. A higher tear breakup time indicates tear film instability.

2.5. Statistical Analysis

Meta-analysis was performed using the Comprehensive Meta-Analysis software, version 3 (Biostat, Englewood, NJ, USA). First, we calculated the standardised mean differences (SMDs) of each index between the post-FLACS time points and baseline. The SMD from each study was computed by dividing the mean difference between each time point and baseline by the standard deviation in order to ensure that the difference was on the same scale. Then, the SMDs were pooled to derive the overall differences between post-FLACS and baseline according to each time point. Second, we compared the differences between the FLACS and MCS groups. The SMDs from each study were pooled to derive the overall values using a similar algorithm. Thus, we could then know which surgery was favoured. The heterogeneity among the studies was determined using the I^2 statistic, and an I^2 statistic of $\geq 50\%$ would represent high heterogeneity. Funnel plots and Egger's test were used to assess publication bias.

3. Results

3.1. Search Results

The PRISMA flow diagram is shown in Figure 1. A total of 67 studies were identified initially. After eliminating duplicated articles ($n = 8$), we removed non-relevant studies by screening titles and abstracts ($n = 52$). Then, a full-text review was performed. Conference abstracts were excluded ($n = 1$). Finally, six studies were enrolled in our meta-analysis [22–27].

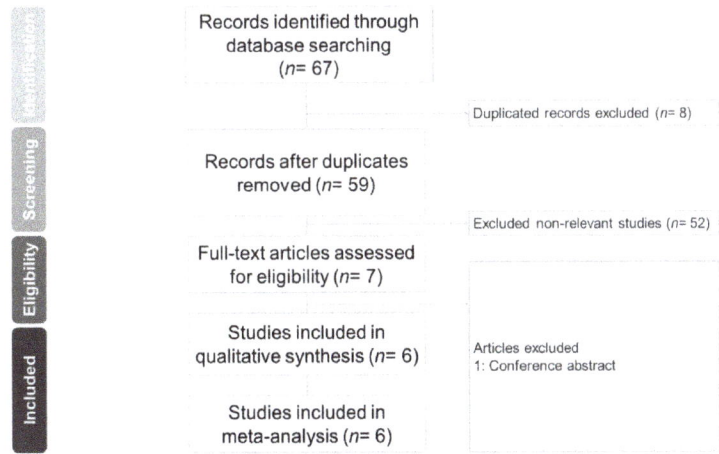

Figure 1. Preferred reporting items for systemic reviews and meta-analyses (PRISM) flow diagram for searching and identifying included studies.

3.2. Evaluation of the Quality of Included Studies

Risk of bias for each study assessed by the ROBINS-I tool is presented in Table 1. The overall results showed that one study (Schargus) had low risk of bias, four studies (Yu, Shao, Zhou, and Xu) had moderate risk of bias, and one study (Ju) had severe risk of bias. None of them had critical risk of bias.

Table 1. Risk of bias assessment for the individual studies included in the meta-analysis.

	D1	D2	D3	D4	D5	D6	D7	Overall
Yu [22]	Moderate	Low	Low	Low	Low	Moderate	Low	Moderate
Shao [23]	Low	Low	Low	Low	Low	Moderate	Moderate	Moderate
Schargus [24]	Low	Low	Low	Low	Low	Low	Low	Low
Ju [25]	Moderate	Low	Low	Low	Severe	Moderate	Moderate	Severe
Zhou [26]	Moderate	Low	Low	Low	Low	Moderate	Moderate	Moderate
Xu [27]	Moderate	Low	Low	Low	Low	Moderate	Moderate	Moderate

D1 = Bias due to confounding; D2 = bias in selection of participants into the study; D3 = bias in classification of interventions; D4 = bias due to deviations from intended interventions; D5 = bias due to missing data; D6 = bias in measurement of outcomes; D7 = bias in selection of the reported result; Low = low risk of bias; Moderate = moderate risk of bias; and Severe = severe risk of bias.

3.3. Characteristics of Included Studies

The characteristics of the studies included in the meta-analysis are presented in Table 2. A total of 678 eyes from 611 patients were enrolled in six studies, with 359 eyes receiving FLACS and 319 eyes receiving MCS. Of the included studies, two were randomised controlled trials and four were prospective cohort studies. Five studies were conducted in China, whereas one study was performed in Germany. The mean age of the participants was 60 to 70 years in most studies.

Table 2. Characteristics of the studies included in meta-analysis.

Author	Year	Type	Country	Study Population	Num of Patients	Num of Eyes	Age, Year (Mean ± SD)	Male (n, %)	Cataract Grading	Phaco Time (s)
Yu [22]	2015	PCS	China	FLACS	73	73	69.0 ± 10.6	34 (46.6)	NS 1+ (24.7%), NS 2+ (53.4%), NS 3+ (17.8%), NS 4+ (4.1%)	35.5 ± 18.4
				MCS	64	64	71.8 ± 10.1	27 (42.2)	NS 1+ (23.4%), NS 2+ (54.7%), NS 3+ (18.8%), NS 4+ (3.1%)	46.7 ± 26.7
Shao [23]	2018	RCT	China	FLACS	123	150	65.7 ± 11.8	67 (44.7)	NR	NR
				MCS	110	150	69.1 ± 12.6	62 (41.3)	NR	NR
Schargus [24]	2020	RCT	Germany	FLACS	17	17	67.4 ± 9.7	7 (41.2)	NR	NR
				MCS	17	17	66.0 ± 7.5	9 (52.9)	NR	NR
Ju [25]	2019	PCS	China	FLACS	38	38	72.6 ± 8.7	16 (42.1)	NR	NR
Zhou [26]	2018	PCS	China	FLACS	26	26	63.2 ± 8.6	11 (42.3)	NS 1+ (0%), NS 2+ (38.5%), NS 3+ (61.5%), NS 4+ (0%)	NR
				MCS	27	27	60.6 ± 6.4	10 (37.0)	NS 1+ (0%), NS 2+ (40.7%), NS 3+ (59.3%), NS 4+ (0%)	NR
Xu [27]	2019	PCS	China	FLACS	55	55	64.5 ± 7.6	25 (45.5)	NS 1+ (36.4%), NS 2+ (36.4%), NS 3+ (30.9%), NS 4+ (12.7%)	37.7 ± 10.5
				MCS	61	61	63.2 ± 8.6	27 (44.3)	NS 1+ (23.0%), NS 2+ (34.4%), NS 3+ (31.1%), NS 4+ (11.5%)	48.0 ± 13.6

Num= number; PCS= prospective cohort study; RCT= randomised controlled trial randomised control trial; FLACS= femto-second laser cataract surgery; MCS = manual cataract surgery; NS = nuclear sclerotic cataract; NR = not reported; and Phaco = phacoemulsification.

3.4. Outcome Assessment of FLACS Group

Table 3 presents the three parameters (OSDI, tear meniscus height, and Schirmer's test) at baseline and postoperative time points. Table 4 shows the values of the other three parameters (fluorescein staining, first tear breakup time, and average tear breakup time). The postoperative time points include day one, week one, one month, and three months.

Table 3. Post-operative changes in OSDI, tear meniscus height, and Schirmer's test.

Study	Group	Num of Eyes	OSDI					Tear Meniscus Height					Schirmer's Test				
			Baseline	1 Day	1 Week	1 Month	3 Months	Baseline	1 Day	1 Week	1 Month	3 Month	Baseline	1 Day	1 Week	1 Month	3 Months
Yu [22]	FLACS	73	22.9 ± 4.2	NR	11.0 ± 5.5	9.1 ± 6.0	NR	0.25 ± 0.12	0.32 ± 0.19	0.27 ± 0.13	0.28 ± 0.16	NR	9.2 ± 7.0	10.3 ± 8.5	7.2 ± 6.4	7.6 ± 7.2	NR
	MCS	64	23.7 ± 5.8	NR	8.8 ± 4.9	8.0 ± 4.9	NR	0.24 ± 0.15	0.30 ± 0.17	0.25 ± 0.15	0.26 ± 0.14	NR	9.4 ± 7.4	11.0 ± 8.6	7.3 ± 6.3	8.6 ± 6.9	NR
Shao [23]	FLACS	150	0.5 ± 0.2	5.3 ± 0.5	5.0 ± 0.5	2.2 ± 0.7	0.6 ± 0.3	0.37 ± 0.09	0.41 ± 0.13	0.22 ± 0.07	0.32 ± 0.05	0.36 ± 0.07	10.9 ± 4.1	11.3 ± 4.9	7.6 ± 3.7	8.8 ± 2.6	11.2 ± 5.0
	MCS	150	0.5 ± 0.4	4.0 ± 0.3	3.5 ± 0.6	1.8 ± 0.7	0.5 ± 0.4	0.35 ± 0.08	0.44 ± 0.11	0.20 ± 0.06	0.30 ± 0.06	0.37 ± 0.06	9.4 ± 4.0	10.7 ± 3.7	7.2 ± 3.3	8.0 ± 2.7	10.1 ± 5.4
Schargus [24]	FLACS	17	NR	NR	NR	NR	NR	NR	NR	NR	NR	NR	13.5 ± 7.9	NR	NR	12.3 ± 7.9	12.0 ± 8.3
	MCS	17	NR	NR	NR	NR	NR	NR	NR	NR	NR	NR	12.7 ± 8.2	NR	NR	14.9 ± 8.2	17.2 ± 8.7
Ju [25]	FLACS	38	8.4 ± 2.1	17.5 ± 5.5	16.0 ± 6.7	13.5 ± 3.6	11.7 ± 3.0	0.32 ± 0.11	0.41 ± 0.13	0.31 ± 0.07	0.30 ± 0.09	0.29 ± 0.07	12.9 ± 3.2	13.4 ± 2.6	10.6 ± 2.3	11.4 ± 3.0	11.6 ± 2.6
Zhou [26]	FLACS	26	NR	NR	NR	NR	NR	NR	NR	NR	NR	NR	12.8 ± 1.9	NR	12.1 ± 1.5	12.2 ± 2.2	12.2 ± 1.7
	MCS	27	NR	NR	NR	NR	NR	NR	NR	NR	NR	NR	13.5 ± 2.5	NR	11.9 ± 1.5	11.3 ± 1.4	13.0 ± 2.1
Xu [27]	FLACS	55	24.5 ± 6.5	NR	10.4 ± 4.2	7.8 ± 4.4	NR	NR	NR	NR	NR	NR	9.4 ± 4.8	NR	9.4 ± 4.0	8.9 ± 3.7	NR
	MCS	61	24.8 ± 7.5	NR	11.6 ± 5.6	8.2 ± 4.9	NR	NR	NR	NR	NR	NR	8.7 ± 4.4	NR	8.7 ± 3.5	8.7 ± 3.3	NR

All data are displayed as mean ± SD. Num = number; OSDI = ocular surface disease index; FLACS = femtosecond laser-assisted cataract surgery; MCS = manual cataract surgery; and NR = not reported.

Table 4. Post-operative changes in fluorescein staining, and tear breakup time.

Study	Group	Num of Eyes	Fluorescein Staining					First Tear Breakup Time					Average Tear Breakup Time				
			Baseline	1 Day	1 Week	1 Month	3 Months	Baseline	1 Day	1 Week	1 Month	3 Month	Baseline	1 Day	1 Week	1 Month	3 Months
Yu [22]	FLACS	73	0.40 ± 0.52	1.46 ± 0.73	0.84 ± 0.53	0.59 ± 0.55	NR	5.5 ± 3.5	4.9 ± 3.4	4.4 ± 2.8	5.6 ± 3.9	NR	7.4 ± 4.3	7.2 ± 4.2	6.5 ± 3.3	7.7 ± 4.5	NR
	MCS	64	0.36 ± 0.49	1.13 ± 0.70	0.67 ± 0.65	0.39 ± 0.55	NR	5.0 ± 2.8	4.7 ± 3.5	4.6 ± 4.0	4.8 ± 3.4	NR	6.8 ± 4.3	7.1 ± 4.2	6.3 ± 4.6	7.1 ± 4.6	NR
Shao [23]	FLACS	150	0.46 ± 0.20	2.34 ± 0.31	1.88 ± 0.29	0.97 ± 0.20	0.51 ± 0.69	11.8 ± 0.8	8.5 ± 1.4	8.0 ± 1.4	11.7 ± 2.1	11.8 ± 2.8	12.7 ± 1.1	10.0 ± 0.8	9.0 ± 0.9	12.6 ± 1.7	12.9 ± 1.6
	MCS	150	0.38 ± 0.22	1.22 ± 0.28	1.02 ± 0.21	0.48 ± 0.14	0.46 ± 0.35	11.0 ± 1.2	8.2 ± 0.0	8.1 ± 1.1	10.9 ± 1.6	11.0 ± 2.1	13.2 ± 1.3	10.1 ± 0.8	9.3 ± 0.9	13.2 ± 1.8	13.4 ± 1.4
Schargus [24]	FLACS	17	5.14 ± 0.39	NR	NR	NR	NR	NR	NR	NR	NR	NR	NR	NR	NR	NR	NR
	MCS	17	5.57 ± 0.17	NR	NR	NR	NR	NR	NR	NR	NR	NR	NR	NR	NR	NR	NR
Ju [25]	FLACS	38	0.89 ± 0.73	4.13 ± 1.17	3.21 ± 0.91	1.34 ± 0.71	1.10 ± 0.77	10.7 ± 1.2	8.1 ± 1.2	7.0 ± 1.7	10.4 ± 1.5	11.1 ± 2.1	11.6 ± 1.0	9.4 ± 1.0	8.5 ± 0.9	11.3 ± 0.8	11.3 ± 0.9
Zhou [26]	FLACS	26	NR	NR	NR	NR	NR	14.3 ± 2.0	NR	10.2 ± 2.5	10.7 ± 2.0	14.2 ± 1.9	NR	NR	NR	NR	NR
	MCS	27	NR	NR	NR	NR	NR	14.4 ± 2.2	NR	8.8 ± 2.0	9.3 ± 1.9	14.3 ± 1.5	NR	NR	NR	NR	NR
Xu [27]	FLACS	55	0.55 ± 0.72	NR	1.38 ± 0.97	0.93 ± 1.02	NR	6.2 ± 2.0	NR	3.6 ± 1.6	4.8 ± 2.1	NR	NR	NR	NR	NR	NR
	MCS	61	0.51 ± 0.52	NR	1.01 ± 0.86	0.66 ± 0.89	NR	6.0 ± 1.6	NR	4.5 ± 2.0	4.8 ± 1.9	NR	NR	NR	NR	NR	NR

All data are displayed as mean ± SD. Num = number; FLACS = femtosecond laser-assisted cataract surgery; MCS = manual cataract surgery; and NR = not reported.

The FLACS group pooled analyses comparing the postoperative and baseline values of the six parameters are presented in Figures 2 and 3. The overall SMDs showed increased values at postoperative day one in four of the six parameters (OSDI, tear meniscus height, Schirmer's test, and fluorescein staining). The increase was statistically significant in tear meniscus height (SMD: 0.456, 95% confidence interval (CI): 0.257 to 0.655), Schirmer's test (SMD: 0.132, 95% CI: 0.037 to 0.226) and fluorescein staining (SMD: 3.550, 95% CI: 0.354 to 6.747), but was not statistically significant in OSDI (SMD: 5.610, 95% CI: −2.191 to 13.411). Subsequently, tear meniscus height and Schirmer's test scores decreased to a level lower than baseline, while OSDI and fluorescein staining scores remained higher than baseline. The SMDs of each parameter had a tendency toward zero over time.

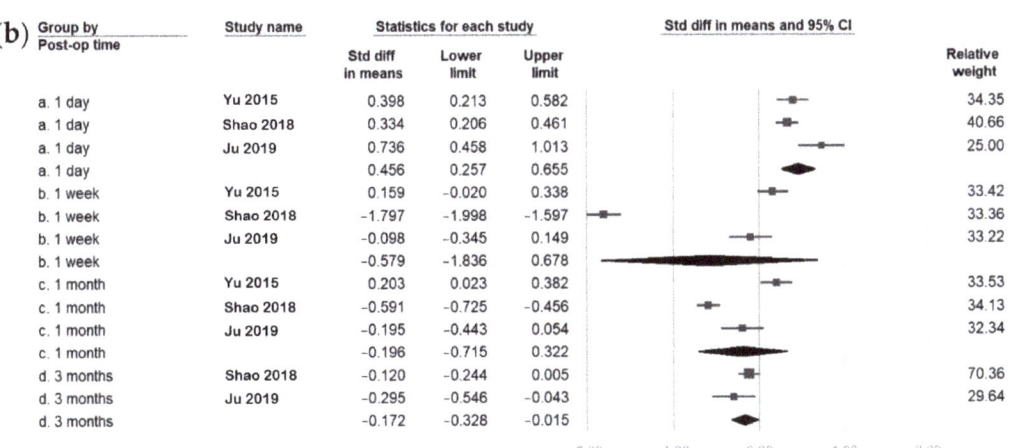

Figure 2. Cont.

(c)

Group by Post-op time	Study name	Std diff in means	Lower limit	Upper limit		Relative weight
a. 1 day	Yu 2015	0.207	0.027	0.386		27.66
a. 1 day	Shao 2018	0.087	-0.037	0.211		57.83
a. 1 day	Ju 2019	0.167	-0.081	0.415		14.50
a. 1 day		0.132	0.037	0.226		
b. 1 week	Yu 2015	-0.350	-0.533	-0.167		20.71
b. 1 week	Shao 2018	-0.840	-0.984	-0.696		21.21
b. 1 week	Ju 2019	-0.779	-1.061	-0.498		19.10
b. 1 week	Zhou 2018	-0.397	-0.706	-0.087		18.58
b. 1 week	Xu 2019	0.000	-0.205	0.205		20.40
b. 1 week		-0.473	-0.808	-0.139		
c. 1 month	Yu 2015	-0.288	-0.470	-0.107		19.50
c. 1 month	Shao 2018	-0.553	-0.686	-0.420		21.90
c. 1 month	Schargus 2020	-0.152	-0.522	0.218		11.12
c. 1 month	Ju 2019	-0.482	-0.743	-0.222		15.58
c. 1 month	Zhou 2018	-0.288	-0.592	0.016		13.64
c. 1 month	Xu 2019	-0.112	-0.318	0.093		18.27
c. 1 month		-0.329	-0.493	-0.165		
d. 3 months	Shao 2018	0.064	-0.060	0.188		30.48
d. 3 months	Schargus 2020	-0.185	-0.556	0.186		20.67
d. 3 months	Ju 2019	-0.435	-0.693	-0.178		25.45
d. 3 months	Zhou 2018	-0.330	-0.636	-0.025		23.40
d. 3 months		-0.207	-0.487	0.074		

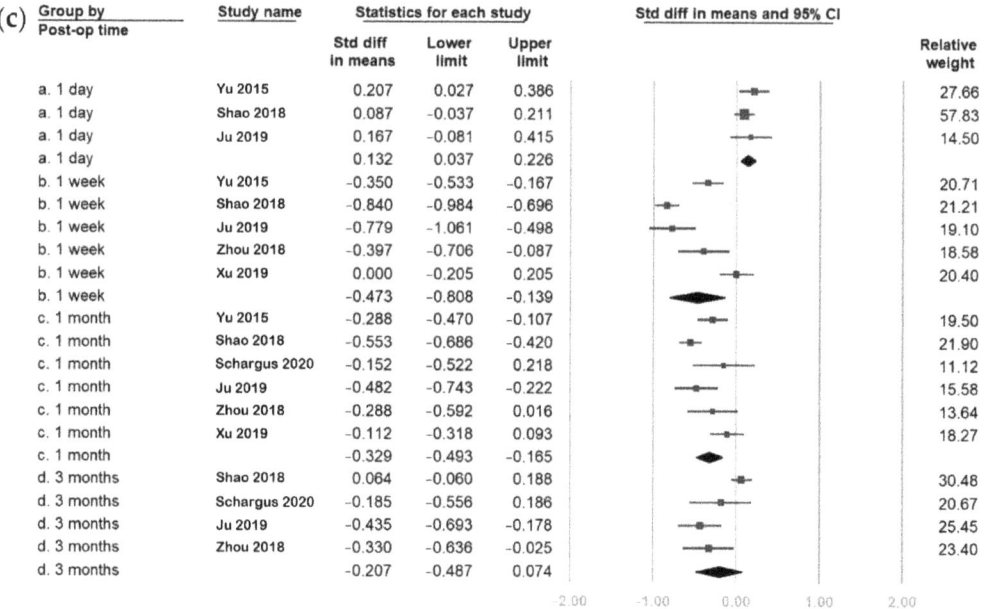

Figure 2. Overall effect of femtosecond laser-assisted cataract surgery (FLACS) on (**a**) ocular surface disease index (OSDI), (**b**) tear meniscus height, and (**c**) Schirmer's test. The square represents the standardised mean difference of each study. The size of square stands for the relative weight of each study. The lozenge represents the overall standardised mean difference.

(a)

Group by Post-op time	Study name	Std diff in means	Lower limit	Upper limit		Relative weight
a. 1 day	Yu 2015	1.130	0.902	1.357		33.54
a. 1 day	Shao 2018	6.559	5.970	7.147		33.22
a. 1 day	Ju 2019	2.987	2.411	3.562		33.24
a. 1 day		3.550	0.354	6.747		
b. 1 week	Yu 2015	0.550	0.359	0.740		25.26
b. 1 week	Shao 2018	5.310	4.829	5.792		24.83
b. 1 week	Ju 2019	2.737	2.201	3.274		24.71
b. 1 week	Xu 2019	0.926	0.682	1.171		25.20
b. 1 week		2.367	0.671	4.064		
c. 1 month	Yu 2015	0.237	0.057	0.418		25.14
c. 1 month	Shao 2018	2.550	2.294	2.806		24.93
c. 1 month	Ju 2019	0.625	0.355	0.894		24.88
c. 1 month	Xu 2019	0.404	0.191	0.617		25.05
c. 1 month		0.952	-0.038	1.942		
d. 3 months	Shao 2018	0.068	-0.056	0.192		62.48
d. 3 months	Ju 2019	0.292	0.040	0.543		37.52
d. 3 months		0.152	-0.060	0.364		

Figure 3. *Cont.*

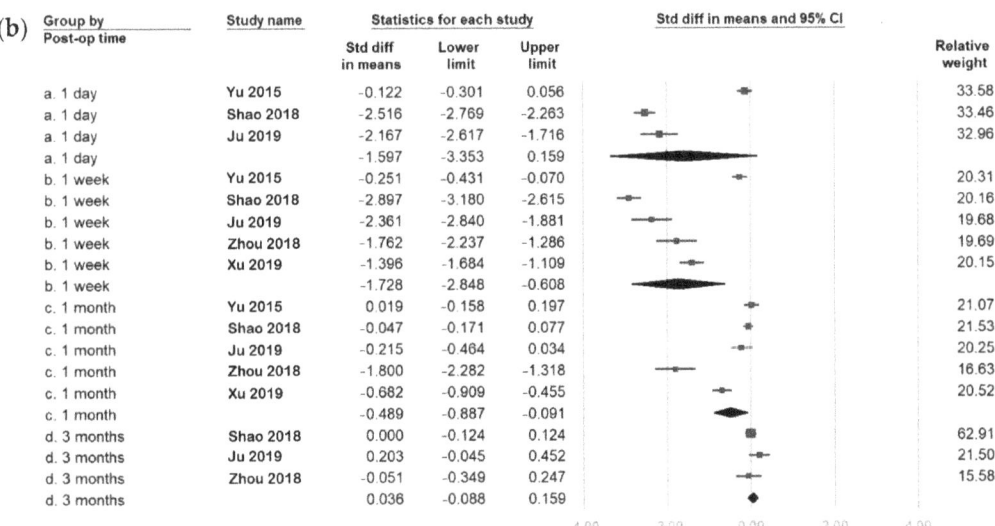

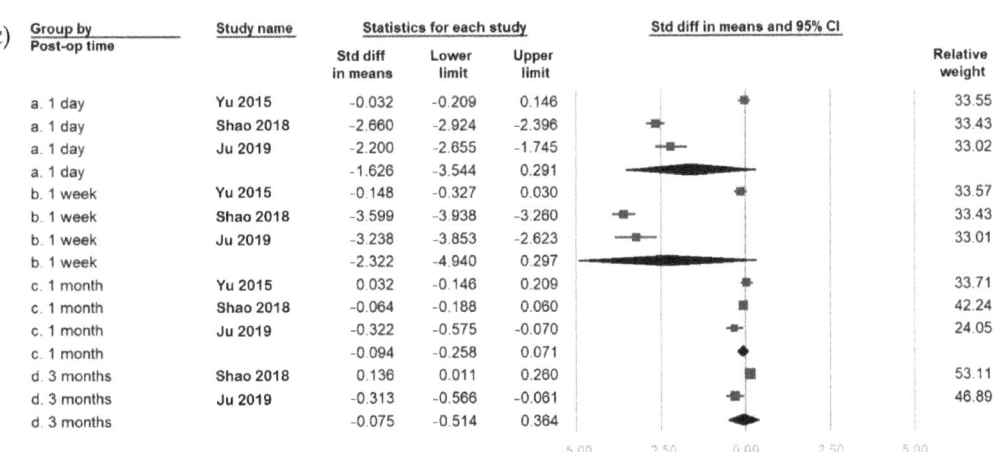

Figure 3. Overall effect of femtosecond laser-assisted cataract surgery (FLACS) on (**a**) fluorescein staining, (**b**) first tear breakup time (fBUT), and (**c**) average tear breakup time (avBUT). The square represents the standardised mean difference of each study. The size of square stands for the relative weight of each study. The lozenge represents the overall standardised mean difference.

Regarding the first and average tear breakup times, both had lower values than baseline from postoperative day one to the first month. The decreased values were only significant in the first tear breakup time at postoperative week one and the first month. The SMDs of the first and average tear breakup times trended towards zero with time. Finally, at postoperative three months, the six parameters were nearly similar to their baseline values except for tear meniscus height, which was significantly lower than at baseline (SMD: −0.172, 95% CI: −0.328 to −0.015).

3.5. Outcome Assessment Comparing FLACS and MCS Group

Figures 4 and 5 compare the postoperative change in six parameters between FLACS and MCS at various postoperative time points. The FLACS group had a higher reduction in tear meniscus height, Schirmer's test, fBUT, and avBUT. In addition, it had a higher increase in OSDI and fluorescent staining than the MCS group at every postoperative time point. In addition, the FLACS group showed less tear secretion postoperatively. However, most differences between FLACS and MCS were becoming less from postoperative day one to three months. Further, the differences were only significant at the following three time points: Schirmer's test at postoperative day one (SMD: −0.208, 95% CI: −0.397 to −0.020), one month (SMD: −0.309, 95% CI: −0.534 to −0.085), and first tear breakup time at postoperative week one (SMD: −0.685, 95% CI: −1.058 to −0.311).

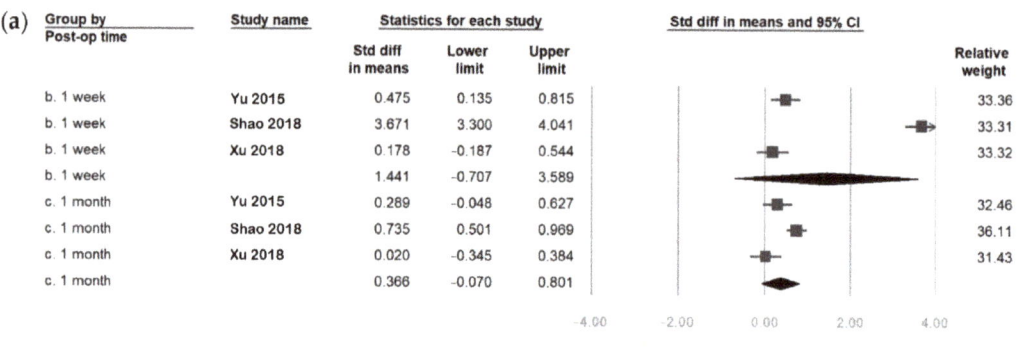

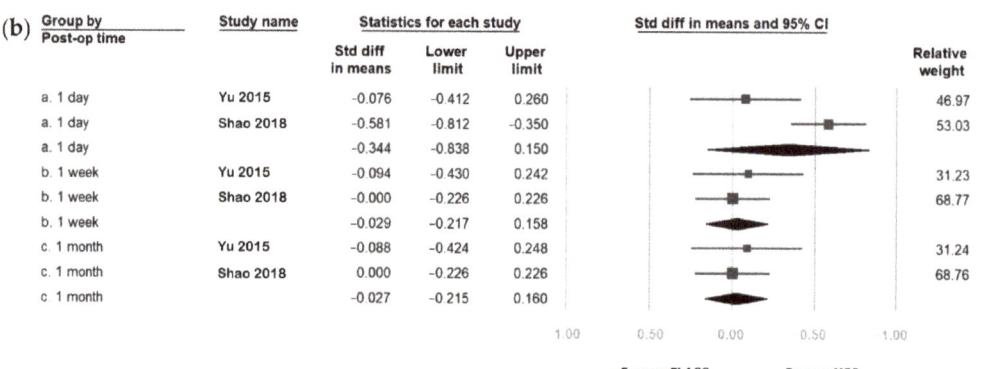

Figure 4. Cont.

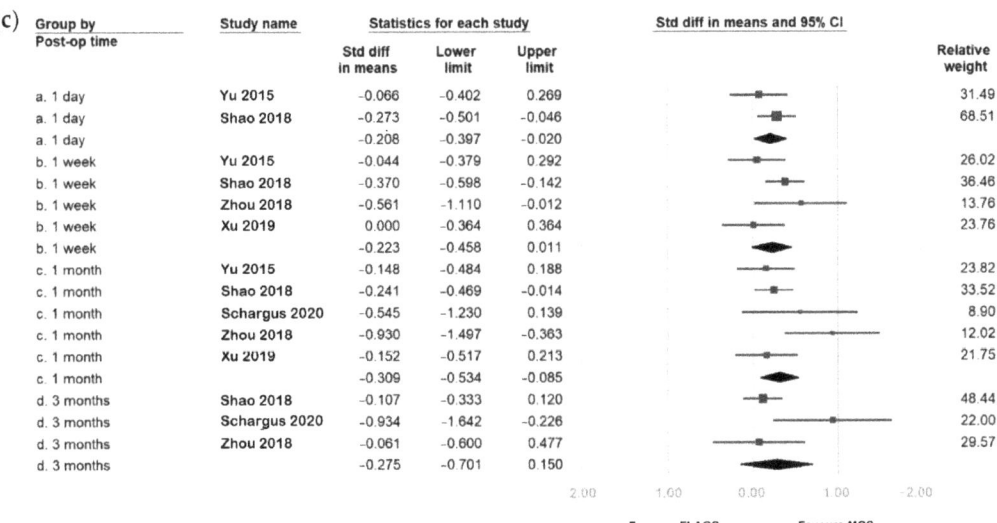

Figure 4. Comparison of (**a**) ocular surface disease index (OSDI), (**b**) tear meniscus height, and (**c**) Schirmer's test between the femtosecond laser-assisted cataract surgery (FLACS) group and manual cataract surgery (MCS) group. I^2 represents heterogeneity. The square represents the standardised mean difference of each study. The size of square stands for the relative weight of each study. The lozenge represents the overall standardised mean difference.

Figure 5. Cont.

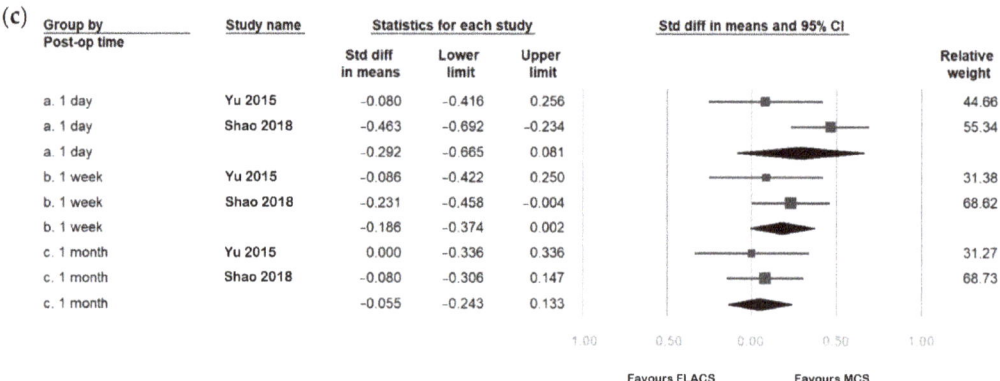

Figure 5. Comparison of (**a**) fluorescein staining, (**b**) first tear breakup time (fBUT), and (**c**) average tear breakup time (avBUT) between the femtosecond laser-assisted cataract surgery (FLACS) group and manual cataract surgery (MCS) group. I^2 represents heterogeneity. The square represents the standardised mean difference of each study. The size of square stands for the relative weight of each study. The lozenge represents the overall standardised mean difference.

3.6. Heterogeneity and Publication Bias

Most analyses showed high between-study heterogeneity when evaluating the SMDs of six parameters ($I^2 > 75\%$). Concerning publication bias, Figure 6 demonstrates the funnel plots of studies regarding the post-FLACS effects. Regarding OSDI, tear meniscus height and Schirmer's test, the p-values of the Egger's test were 0.31, 0.94, and 0.65, respectively—revealing no significant publication biases. Significant publication biases were noted regarding post-FLACS effects corresponding to fluorescent staining, first tear breakup time, and average breakup time (all Egger's tests $p < 0.01$).

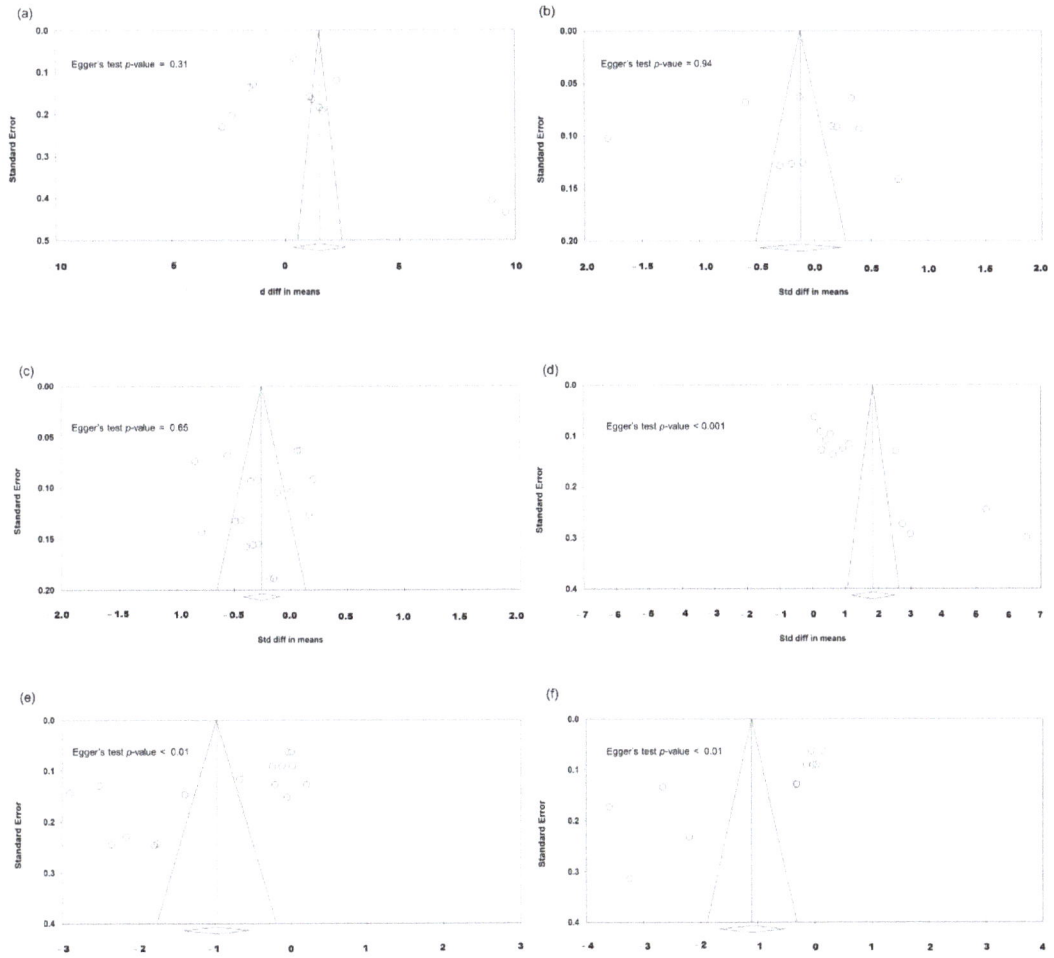

Figure 6. Funnel plots evaluating the publication biases regarding post-FLACS impacts on the six dry eye parameters (**a**) OSDI, (**b**) tear meniscus height, (**c**) Schirmer's test, (**d**) fluorescein staining, (**e**) fBUT, and (**f**) avBUT. The lozenge stands for overall standardised mean difference.

Funnel plots of the studies comparing postoperative effects between FLACS and MCS are presented in Figure 7. They exhibited no significant publication biases in all six parameters of dry eye symptoms/signs (all Egger's tests $p > 0.1$).

Since the publication bias is statistically significant regarding post-FLACS impacts on fluorescein staining, fBUT, and avBUT, we applied the trim-and-fill method to deal with the publication biases. After trimming the studies that caused a funnel plot's asymmetry and filling imputed missing studies in the funnel plot based on the bias-corrected overall estimate, the funnel plots were adjusted and are presented in Figure 8. The direction and significance of SMD did not change after adjusting the publication biases. Therefore, our previous statistical analyses regarding SMD were convincible.

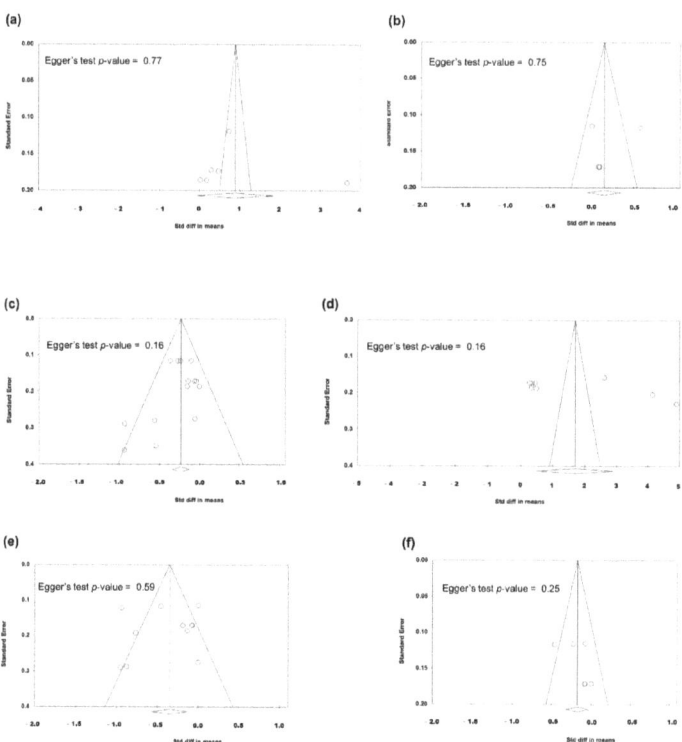

Figure 7. Funnel plots evaluating the publication biases regarding the comparison between FLACS and MCS on the six dry eye parameters (**a**) OSDI, (**b**) tear meniscus height, (**c**) Schirmer's test, (**d**) fluorescein staining, (**e**) fBUT, and (**f**) avBUT. The lozenge stands for overall standardised mean difference.

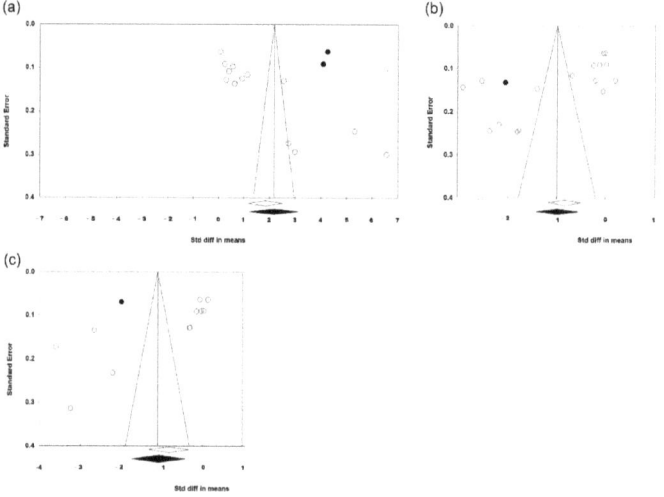

Figure 8. Funnel plots after using trim-and-fill method to adjust the publication biases regarding post-FLACS impacts on the dry eye parameters (**a**) fluorescein staining, (**b**) fBUT, and (**c**) avBUT. The lozenge stands for overall standardised mean difference. The data points for imputed studies are highlighted in black.

4. Discussion

This meta-analysis included six studies focusing on dry eye after FLACS. Six parameters (OSDI, tear meniscus height, Schirmer's test, fluorescein staining, first breakup time, and average breakup time) were used to evaluate dry eye symptoms/signs, which were also compared between FLACS and MCS groups. On postoperative day one, eyes receiving FLACS had transiently increased dry eye symptoms (OSDI) and tear secretion (tear meniscus height and Schirmer's test) but then decreased. Microscopic ocular surface damage (fluorescein staining) was significantly increased on postoperative day one and week one but improved after one month. Tear film instability (first breakup time and average breakup time) lasted for one month after surgery and then returned to the baseline level. Three months after surgery, only tear meniscus height was significantly decreased, while all the other parameters were similar to baseline. Compared with MCS, FLACS had a greater tendency towards dry eye in the early postoperative stage. However, the dry eye symptoms/signs between FLACS and MCS showed no significant differences three months after surgery.

This study is the first meta-analysis to compare the impact on postoperative dry eye between FLACS and MCS, to the best of our knowledge. In our study, a transient increase in tear secretion on postoperative day one may be related to surgical-induced pain. One possible explanation for the tear film instability presenting itself immediately after surgery is inflammation. Wound epithelial cells secrete inflammatory factors that accumulate in tears. The bandage of the eye decreases the tear removal rate and aggravates the inflammatory reaction, hyperosmolarity in tears, and subjective discomfort.

Regarding microscopic ocular surface damage, multiple reasons are responsible, including preoperative instillation of povidone-iodine and local anaesthesia [28,29], intraoperative irrigation, and light exposure [30]. Dry eye symptoms improved, but signs were worse at postoperative week one, implying more cytokines were released from the wound in order to induce inflammation. In addition, our study found that FLACS had a more severe effect on dry eye than MCS. This effect may be due to the suction ring in FLACS, injuring the limbal stem cells, conjunctival epithelium, and goblet cells. It is similar to the dry eye mechanism after laser-assisted in situ keratomileusis [31]. In addition, the extra laser procedure in FLACS leads to prolonged light exposure, thereby deteriorating tear film stability.

Fortunately, in our study, the symptoms/signs of dry eye immediately following FLACS almost returned to baseline within three months postoperatively. This result might be explained by the anti-inflammatory effects of postoperative eye drops. Previous studies have revealed that neuroregeneration occurs 25 days postoperatively [32], supporting our finding that postoperative dry eye tends to improve. Furthermore, the differences in dry eye parameters between FLACS and MCS mainly have no significant difference and have a decreasing trend. However, Yu et al. have found that FLACS causes more ocular surface damage than MCS in patients with pre-existing dry eye [22]. Therefore, preoperative screening and postoperative treatment for dry eye should be performed meticulously for those receiving FLACS with a pre-existing unhealthy ocular surface.

The main limitation of our meta-analysis is the heterogeneity among the included studies. The between-study variations may arise from differences in surgical machines, study protocols, inclusion criteria, and perioperative use of topical medication. Five of the six enrolled studies used the LenSx femtosecond laser system (Alcon Laboratories, Fort Worth, TX, USA). Only Schargus et al. used the CATALYS laser system (Johnson and Johnson, New Brunswick, NJ, USA). Different docking devices used in the laser platforms may cause different effects on the ocular surface [24,33]. Another limitation is that most included studies have a non-randomised design, increasing bias.

Moreover, the parameters used in our meta-analysis (OSDI, tear meniscus height, Schirmer's test, fluorescein staining, and tear breakup time) are not objective enough and are prone to observers' errors. Previous studies have suggested that tear film osmolarity and matrix metalloproteinase levels are more reliable dry eye tests and correlate well with dry eye severity [20,34,35]. In addition, meibomian gland dysfunction, lipid layer thickness, inflammatory levels, and goblet cell densities also play an important role in dry eye [36,37]. These parameters should be assessed in further studies. Still another limitation is that we cannot perform subgroup analyses according to cataract grading or phacoemulsification time, which are relevant with post-operative dry eye. We have extracted data of cataract grading from three studies (Yu, Zhou, and Xu) and phacoemulsification time from two studies (Yu and Xu). However, the information was presented as overall proportion or mean, without mentioning the individual dry eye symptoms/signs corresponding to each category of cataract grading or phacoemulsification time. The lack of details and the too few study numbers makes subgroup analyses infeasible.

The strength of our study is that our results provide an evaluation of dry eye symptoms/signs following FLACS and include comparisons with those following MCS. Therefore, we could have a better understanding of postoperative dry eye risk. More comprehensive studies will need to be conducted, thereby supplying evidence for further meta-analyses.

5. Conclusions

In conclusion, both FLACS and MCS can induce dry eye. The adverse effects of FLACS on the ocular surface are more severe in FLACS than in MCS. Fortunately, these effects are transient and are resolved within three months after surgery. Cataract surgeons should select FLACS candidates carefully and adopt preoperative evaluation and postoperative therapy for dry eye. Further studies are warranted to verify and understand the post-FLACS dry eye mechanism.

Author Contributions: Conceptualisation, Y.-Y.C.; methodology, Y.-Y.C.; validation, W.-T.C., Y.-Y.C. and M.-C.H.; formal analysis, W.-T.C., Y.-Y.C. and M.-C.H.; investigation, W.-T.C. and Y.-Y.C.; resources, Y.-Y.C.; writing—original draft preparation, W.-T.C.; writing—review and editing, Y.-Y.C.; visualisation, Y.-Y.C. and M.-C.H.; funding acquisition, Y.-Y.C. All authors have read and agreed to the published version of the manuscript.

Funding: This work was supported by the Taichung Veterans General Hospital (grant number: TCVGH-1116901B).

Institutional Review Board Statement: This is a meta-analysis study. The Taichung Veterans General Hospital Research Ethics Committee have confirmed that no ethical approval is required.

Informed Consent Statement: This is a meta-analysis study. The informed consent is not applicable.

Data Availability Statement: The data from this study are available on request from the corresponding author.

Acknowledgments: We would like to acknowledge Taichung Veterans General Hospital for their database resources.

Conflicts of Interest: The authors declare no conflict of interest. The funders had no role in the design of the study, nor in the collection, analyses, or interpretation of data. Neither did they have a role in the writing of the manuscript, nor in the decision to publish the results.

References

1. Zamora, M.G.; Caballero, E.F.; Maldonado, M.J. Short-term changes in ocular surface signs and symptoms after phacoemulsification. *Eur. J. Ophthalmol.* **2020**, *30*, 1301–1307. [CrossRef]
2. Lu, Q.; Lu, Y.; Zhu, X. Dry eye and phacoemulsification cataract surgery: A systematic review and meta-analysis. *Front. Med.* **2021**, *8*, 649030. [CrossRef] [PubMed]
3. Kasetsuwan, N.; Satitpitakul, V.; Changul, T.; Jariyakosol, S. Incidence and pattern of dry eye after cataract surgery. *PLoS ONE* **2013**, *8*, e78657. [CrossRef]
4. Li, X.M.; Hu, L.; Hu, J.; Wang, W. Investigation of dry eye disease and analysis of the pathogenic factors in patients after cataract surgery. *Cornea* **2007**, *26*, S16–S20. [CrossRef] [PubMed]
5. Khanal, S.; Tomlinson, A.; Esakowitz, L.; Bhatt, P.; Jones, D.; Nabili, S.; Mukerji, S. Changes in corneal sensitivity and tear physiology after phacoemulsification. *Ophthalmic Physiol. Opt. J. Br. Coll. Ophthalmic Opt. Optom.* **2008**, *28*, 127–134. [CrossRef] [PubMed]

8. Oh, T.; Jung, Y.; Chang, D.; Kim, J.; Kim, H. Changes in the tear film and ocular surface after cataract surgery. *Jpn. J. Ophthalmol.* **2012**, *56*, 113–118. [CrossRef] [PubMed]
9. Park, D.H.; Chung, J.K.; Seo, D.R.; Lee, S.J. Clinical effects and safety of 3% diquafosol ophthalmic solution for patients with dry eye after cataract surgery: A randomized controlled trial. *Am. J. Ophthalmol.* **2016**, *163*, 122–131.e122. [CrossRef] [PubMed]
10. Igarashi, T.; Takahashi, H.; Kobayashi, M.; Kunishige, T.; Arima, T.; Fujimoto, C.; Suzuki, H.; Okuda, T.; Takahashi, H. Changes in tear osmolarity after cataract surgery. *J. Nippon. Med. Sch. Nippon. Ika Daigaku Zasshi* **2021**, *88*, 204–208. [CrossRef]
11. Kolb, C.M.; Shajari, M.; Mathys, L.; Herrmann, E.; Petermann, K.; Mayer, W.J.; Priglinger, S.; Kohnen, T. Comparison of femtosecond laser-assisted cataract surgery and conventional cataract surgery: A meta-analysis and systematic review. *J. Cataract. Refract. Surg.* **2020**, *46*, 1075–1085. [CrossRef] [PubMed]
12. Naderi, K.; Gormley, J.; O'Brart, D. Cataract surgery and dry eye disease: A review. *Eur. J. Ophthalmol.* **2020**, *30*, 840–855. [CrossRef]
13. Chee, S.P.; Yang, Y.; Wong, M.H.Y. Randomized controlled trial comparing femtosecond laser-assisted with conventional phacoemulsification on dense cataracts. *Am. J. Ophthalmol.* **2021**, *229*, 1–7. [CrossRef] [PubMed]
14. Day, A.C.; Burr, J.M.; Bennett, K.; Bunce, C.; Doré, C.J.; Rubin, G.S.; Nanavaty, M.A.; Balaggan, K.S.; Wilkins, M.R. Femtosecond laser-assisted cataract surgery versus phacoemulsification cataract surgery (fact): A randomized noninferiority trial. *Ophthalmology* **2020**, *127*, 1012–1019. [CrossRef] [PubMed]
15. Stanojcic, N.; Roberts, H.W.; Wagh, V.K.; Li, J.O.; Naderi, K.; O'Brart, D.P. A randomised controlled trial comparing femtosecond laser-assisted cataract surgery versus conventional phacoemulsification surgery: 12-month results. *Br. J. Ophthalmol.* **2021**, *105*, 631–638. [CrossRef] [PubMed]
16. Popovic, M.; Campos-Möller, X.; Schlenker, M.B.; Ahmed, I.I.K. Efficacy and safety of femtosecond laser-assisted cataract surgery compared with manual cataract surgery: A meta-analysis of 14,567 eyes. *Ophthalmology* **2016**, *123*, 2113–2126. [CrossRef] [PubMed]
17. Ang, R.E.T.; Quinto, M.M.S.; Cruz, E.M.; Rivera, M.C.R.; Martinez, G.H.A. Comparison of clinical outcomes between femtosecond laser-assisted versus conventional phacoemulsification. *Eye Vis.* **2018**, *5*, 8. [CrossRef] [PubMed]
18. Ferreira, T.B.; Ribeiro, F.J.; Pinheiro, J.; Ribeiro, P.; O'Neill, J.G. Comparison of surgically induced astigmatism and morphologic features resulting from femtosecond laser and manual clear corneal incisions for cataract surgery. *J. Refract. Surg.* **2018**, *34*, 322–329. [CrossRef]
19. Schiffman, R.M.; Christianson, M.D.; Jacobsen, G.; Hirsch, J.D.; Reis, B.L. Reliability and validity of the ocular surface disease index. *Arch. Ophthalmol.* **2000**, *118*, 615–621. [CrossRef]
20. Wei, A.; Le, Q.; Hong, J.; Wang, W.; Wang, F.; Xu, J. Assessment of lower tear meniscus. *Optom. Vis. Sci. Off. Publ. Am. Acad. Optom.* **2016**, *93*, 1420–1425. [CrossRef]
21. Stevens, S. Schirmer's test. *Community Eye Health* **2011**, *24*, 45. [PubMed]
22. Wolffsohn, J.S.; Arita, R.; Chalmers, R.; Djalilian, A.; Dogru, M.; Dumbleton, K.; Gupta, P.K.; Karpecki, P.; Lazreg, S.; Pult, H.; et al. Tfos dews ii diagnostic methodology report. *Ocul. Surf.* **2017**, *15*, 539–574. [CrossRef]
23. Hong, J.; Sun, X.; Wei, A.; Cui, X.; Li, Y.; Qian, T.; Wang, W.; Xu, J. Assessment of tear film stability in dry eye with a newly developed keratograph. *Cornea* **2013**, *32*, 716–721. [CrossRef]
24. Yu, Y.; Hua, H.; Wu, M.; Yu, Y.; Yu, W.; Lai, K.; Yao, K. Evaluation of dry eye after femtosecond laser-assisted cataract surgery. *J. Cataract. Refract. Surg.* **2015**, *41*, 2614–2623. [CrossRef] [PubMed]
25. Shao, D.; Zhu, X.; Sun, W.; Cheng, P.; Chen, W.; Wang, H. Effects of femtosecond laser-assisted cataract surgery on dry eye. *Exp. Ther. Med.* **2018**, *16*, 5073–5078. [CrossRef] [PubMed]
26. Schargus, M.; Ivanova, S.; Stute, G.; Dick, H.B.; Joachim, S.C. Comparable effects on tear film parameters after femtosecond laser-assisted and conventional cataract surgery. *Int. Ophthalmol.* **2020**, *40*, 3097–3104. [CrossRef] [PubMed]
27. Ju, R.H.; Chen, Y.; Chen, H.S.; Zhou, W.J.; Yang, W.; Lin, Z.D.; Wu, Z.M. Changes in ocular surface status and dry eye symptoms following femtosecond laser-assisted cataract surgery. *Int. J. Ophthalmol.* **2019**, *12*, 1122–1126. [CrossRef] [PubMed]
28. Zhou, Y.; Zhang, H. Changes of tear film and corneal sensitivity after femtosecond laser-assisted cataract extraction surgery. *Chin. J. Exp. Ophthalmol.* **2018**, *36*, 222–226.
29. Xu, R.; Zhao, S. The effect comparison of femtosecond laser-assisted phacoemusification and microincision phacoemusification on ocualr surface. *Chin. J. Exp. Ophthalmol.* **2018**, *37*, 907–913.
30. Yanai, R.; Yamada, N.; Ueda, K.; Tajiri, M.; Matsumoto, T.; Kido, K.; Nakamura, S.; Saito, F.; Nishida, T. Evaluation of povidone-iodine as a disinfectant solution for contact lenses: Antimicrobial activity and cytotoxicity for corneal epithelial cells. *Contact Lens Anterior Eye J. Br. Contact Lens Assoc.* **2006**, *29*, 85–91. [CrossRef]
31. Rosenwasser, G.O. Complications of topical ocular anesthetics. *Int. Ophthalmol. Clin.* **1989**, *29*, 153–158. [CrossRef]
32. Hwang, H.B.; Kim, H.S. Phototoxic effects of an operating microscope on the ocular surface and tear film. *Cornea* **2014**, *33*, 82–90. [CrossRef]
33. Salomão, M.Q.; Ambrósio, R., Jr.; Wilson, S.E. Dry eye associated with laser in situ keratomileusis: Mechanical microkeratome versus femtosecond laser. *J. Cataract. Refract. Surg.* **2009**, *35*, 1756–1760. [CrossRef] [PubMed]
34. Shaheen, B.S.; Bakir, M.; Jain, S. Corneal nerves in health and disease. *Surv. Ophthalmol.* **2014**, *59*, 263–285. [CrossRef] [PubMed]
35. Wu, B.M.; Williams, G.P.; Tan, A.; Mehta, J.S. A comparison of different operating systems for femtosecond lasers in cataract surgery. *J. Ophthalmol.* **2015**, *2015*, 616478. [CrossRef] [PubMed]

34. Tomlinson, A.; Khanal, S.; Ramaesh, K.; Diaper, C.; McFadyen, A. Tear film osmolarity: Determination of a referent for dry eye diagnosis. *Investig. Ophthalmol. Vis. Sci.* **2006**, *47*, 4309–4315. [CrossRef] [PubMed]
35. Chotikavanich, S.; de Paiva, C.S.; Li, D.Q.; Chen, J.J.; Bian, F.; Farley, W.J.; Pflugfelder, S.C. Production and activity of matrix metalloproteinase-9 on the ocular surface increase in dysfunctional tear syndrome. *Investig. Ophthalmol. Vis. Sci.* **2009**, *50*, 3203–3209. [CrossRef] [PubMed]
36. Usuba, F.S.; de Medeiros-Ribeiro, A.C.; Novaes, P.; Aikawa, N.E.; Bonfiglioli, K.; Santo, R.M.; Bonfá, E.; Alves, M.R. Dry eye in rheumatoid arthritis patients under tnf-inhibitors: Conjunctival goblet cell as an early ocular biomarker. *Sci. Rep.* **2020**, *10*, 14054. [CrossRef]
37. Kim, W.J.; Ahn, Y.J.; Kim, M.H.; Kim, H.S.; Kim, M.S.; Kim, E.C. Lipid layer thickness decrease due to meibomian gland dysfunction leads to tear film instability and reflex tear secretion. *Ann. Med.* **2022**, *54*, 893–899. [CrossRef]

MDPI
St. Alban-Anlage 66
4052 Basel
Switzerland
Tel. +41 61 683 77 34
Fax +41 61 302 89 18
www.mdpi.com

Journal of Clinical Medicine Editorial Office
E-mail: jcm@mdpi.com
www.mdpi.com/journal/jcm

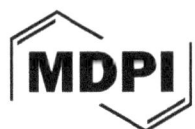

www.ingramcontent.com/pod-product-compliance
Lightning Source LLC
LaVergne TN
LVHW070611100526
838202LV00012B/617